The Complete Guide to
# Natural Medicines

Celia G. Kellett, MRPharm.S

# The Complete Guide to
# Natural Medicines

Index compiled by Ann Griffiths

SAFFRON WALDEN
THE C.W. DANIEL COMPANY LIMITED

First published in 2003 in the United Kingdom by
The C.W. Daniel Company Limited
1 Church Path, Saffron Walden,
Essex CB10 1JP, United Kingdom

ISBN 0 85207 373 9

Designed by Jane Norman
Produced in association with Book Production Consultants, plc,
25–27 High Street, Chesterton, Cambridge CB4 1ND
Typeset by Cambridge Photosetting Services, Cambridge
Printed and bound by St Edmundsbury Press, Bury St Edmunds, Suffolk.

# Acknowledgements

My thanks to all the manufacturers who so kindly responded to my request for information to make this book possible. Especially to Potter's who have allowed me to use their Herbal Cyclopaedia as an information source, also to Weleda for the use of their Natural Medicines Formulary.

# Contents

# Introduction

Although born in Nottingham, I spent most of my childhood living in Prenton on the outskirts of Birkenhead. We lived above my parents' shop and had no garden, only a backyard to play in – so my playground was up the lane, past the duck-pond, to the fields beyond, where I picked wild flowers and blackberries. The wild flowers were taken home to be stuck in a jar of water, or carefully pressed between the pages of whichever big book came to hand. Other older children told me not to pick dandelions as they made you wet the bed – a folklore reference to the diuretic properties of dandelion root. They also showed me that a crushed dock leaf was the treatment for nettle stings – even today I find this treatment more effective than the antihistamine creams you can buy. I remember trying to make perfume by soaking a handful of rose petals in water, but of course they turned brown, and the resulting smelly mess had to be thrown away.

It would be a good few years later that a study of chemistry would reveal that essential oils were soluble in other oils or alcohol, but were not soluble in water, and that a huge quantity of rose petals were needed to produce even a small quantity of oil. For many years I have worked as a community pharmacist, and over that time I have noticed an increasing interest in natural medicines and remedies and in a desire for information about them. This book will, I hope, provide that information.

## Herbal Medicines

Plants have been used as food and as medicine since the dawn of man. The earliest known evidence of text on the subject of medicinal plants is to be found on clay tablets, written by the Sumerians in about 3000 bc. Ancient Egyptian papyri dating from 1500 bc have been found, containing prescriptions using natural products such as caraway, coriander, garlic, linseed, peppermint, figs, fennel, anise, poppy and castor oil. Aristotle and Hippocrates developed theories of medicine which, for 1,500 years, influenced the use of medicinal plants. The Greek botanist and physician Dioscorides (ad 40–90) compiled the first systematic description of nearly 600 plants, their actions and uses. Galen (ad 130–201) further developed this work. Avicenna (ad 980–1037) was a Persian philosopher and physician who wrote many books on medicine, based on the work of Hippocrates, Dioscorides and Galen, which, for several hundred years, became the major textbooks on medicine.

All these books had to be written by hand and it was only with the invention of the printing press by Guttenberg in the mid 15th century that mass production became possible. John Gerard published his *Herball* in 1596 and Nicholas Culpeper published his herbal in 1653 and also published an English translation of the Royal College of Physicians' Latin *Pharmacopeia*, so making it accessible to ordinary people. These books, and others like them, were in common use well into the 19th century.

Herbs frequently have several common names, derived from specific medicinal properties they possess. The Anglo-Saxon word for plant is 'wort', and is still in use today, as in St John's wort, pilewort, coughwort, etc. Latin, Greek, Arabic and other languages are also to be found in the origin of many plant names. The Linnean nomenclature, introduced in the 18th century, uses Latin, and many of these names also have interesting origins.

Herbal medicine, now sometimes called phytotherapy, is currently undergoing a renaissance. Modern analytical techniques have enabled scientists to determine the actual chemical constituents of plants, to test batches of plants to ensure quality control and make possible the standardisation of active ingredients. The soil and climate affect the quality of the plants: rosemary, hyssop, horehound, mint, marjoram, thyme and juniper prefer an alkaline soil; whilst lemon balm, borage and centaury prefer an acid soil. Roman chamomile, coriander, fennel and thyme like sandy soils. Mediterranean herbs produce more oils if grown in soil that is not too rich.

Herbal medicine sometimes uses the whole plant, but often only specific parts are used, such as the leaves, roots, bark, seeds or flowers. Herbal medicines are prepared from the dried plant material, or from extracts of them – a tincture is an alcoholic extract – and in some cases the fresh plants are used. It would appear that the many constituents of the plant are synergistic, that is, they have a greater effect in combination than would be expected of the individual components by themselves.

The overall therapeutic action depends on the combination of the many constituents present in the plant all acting together. The chemically pure substances used in conventional, or allopathic, medicine rarely have the same therapeutic effect as those of the plant material from which they have been obtained. The effects of herbal medicines are gentler, and side effects are rare when taken in the recommended dosage. Some herbal medicines, such as laxatives, have an effect within a few hours, whilst many others take time to achieve their full effect. It may take a month or two of regular use to determine this. Although herbal medicines can generally be taken in conjunction with other medicines, there are exceptions. They can interact with some prescribed medicines: any such problems are mentioned towards the end of each entry in the A–Z section of this book. If you are pregnant or breast-feeding or have any doubt about taking any medicinal product, including herbal medicines, you should consult your pharmacist. If you are considering stopping prescribed medication in favour of a natural medicine, you must first discuss the matter with your doctor.

Potter's has been making herbal medicines since 1812, when Henry Potter opened his herbalist business in London. Now based in Wigan, Lancashire, Potter's is the leading manufacturer of herbal medicines sold to the public, and it also supplies herbal practitioners with fluid extracts, tinctures, galenicals and crude herbs.

Lane's, based in Gloucester, was founded in the early 1920s and is another leading manufacturer of herbal medicines.

## Homoeopathic Medicines

Homoeopathy was developed by Samuel Hahnemann, and his findings were published in a *Materia Medica* in 1810. In homoeopathy, the symptoms of an illness are viewed as a sign of the body's attempt to heal itself. A homoeopathic medicine is selected that is capable of producing similar symptoms in a well person. Thus homoeopathy attempts to stimulate the body's own natural healing capacity, with the homoeopathic remedy acting as a trigger to the body's own ability to heal itself. Homoeopathic medicines generally do not have side effects, because their mode of action is different from conventional medicine. They can be taken alongside conventional (allopathic) medicines. They are safe for children and are generally considered to be safe in pregnancy, although they should only be taken on your doctor's advice.

Nelson's, founded in 1860, is Europe's oldest and the UK's largest manufacturer of homoeopathic medicines. Weleda, founded in Switzerland in 1921, and in the UK since 1925, is the other leading manufacturer of homoeopathic medicines.

## Anthroposophical Medicines

Anthroposophical medicine seeks to extend the benefits of conventional medicine, drawing its inspiration from the work of Rudolph Steiner (1861–1925), whose insights lead to a fuller understanding of man as a unique being, with links to both the universe and the natural world around us. This philosophy refers not only to the ingredients and manufacturing process, but also to the way the medicines work. Anthroposophical medicines make use of man's relationship with the mineral, plant and animal kingdoms from which they are prepared. They base their action on a fourfold understanding of the human body, which explains the interrelationships of the physical body, life force, feelings and ego within the human being. This interaction determines the balance between health and illness. Normally health is maintained by the systems being in harmony. Illness is seen as a result of disharmony, which causes imbalance in the subtle interplay of forces which make up the whole human being. Weleda is the leading manufacturer in this field.

## Allopathic Medicines

Conventional, or allopathic, medicines make up the vast majority of medicines that are bought or prescribed. Many are of natural origin, although perhaps people are not particularly aware of this. Plants have been mankind's main source of medicines since the beginning. Plant-based medicines provide nearly 70% of the world's needs. The majority of modern drugs are now produced synthetically, but many were originally discovered in plants. Even antibiotics originate from moulds. (Country folk knew this, long before Sir Alexander Fleming discovered penicillin.) Even in this new millennium pharmaceutical companies still research plants for suitable compounds that could be used as medicines; for example, the latest medicine for Alzheimer's disease contains galantamine, an alkaloid found in daffodil bulbs.

## Aromatherapy

For thousands of years essential oils* have been used to enhance physical and emotional wellbeing. Essential oils are extracted from herbs, spices, flowers, woods and resins in a variety of methods. Apart from lavender and tea tree, essential oils should never be used undiluted, but should be mixed with a base or carrier oil. Some should not be taken internally. See the A–Z for further information on their use.

## How to use this book

This book is in three parts:

**Part 1** is an A–Z of minerals, plants and a few animals, parts of which are used as medicines. Each entry explains what it is, where it comes from, what it does and what it is used for, with any contraindications that may apply to its use. The herbal entries list numerous uses, some of which may only be applicable to treatment by a herbal practitioner.

**Part 2** is the Product Index, divided into different sections according to symptoms, for example indigestion, cough and colds and slimming, to make products easier to find. All the medicines and remedies listed in the Product Index have product licences, indicated by the PL number on the packaging. A product licence is only granted by the licensing authority, the Medicines Control Agency, with the support of clinical and pharmaceutical data. This means that they conform to strict criteria on purity and safety and they have proved to be effective for the conditions for which they are recommended.

Many other products do not have product licences and are sold as food supplements. Absence of a product licence means that their manufacturers are not allowed to make medicinal claims for such products.

**Part 3** contains a glossary of technical terms, plant and animal indexes, plus other information that may be helpful to the reader.

## Warning

It is not recommended that you collect your own plants for medicinal use, unless you are absolutely sure you have the correct species. Everyone knows what a dandelion* looks like, but do they know the difference between the greater and lesser celandine*? Some plants look very similar to others when in fact they may have totally different actions and uses.

When choosing a medicine or remedy, whether herbal, homoeopathic, anthroposophic or allopathic, ask your pharmacist for advice as to its suitability for you, and give details of any other prescribed medication you may be taking.

If you are ever asked to list the medication you regularly take, for example, if you go into hospital, don't forget to mention any herbal medicines you are taking, as they may affect the treatment you will be receiving there. If you are to undergo surgery, you should be aware that because some herbal medicines and food supplements can cause problems you must tell both the surgeon and the anaesthetist what you are taking. For example garlic*, ginkgo* and ginseng* can all lead to an increased risk of bleeding; echinacea* can cause poor wound-healing and an increased risk of infection; ephedra* can cause a heart attack or stroke with certain anaesthetics; kava kava* and valerian* could increase the sedative effects of anaesthetics; and St John's wort* can interact with other drugs. It would be best to stop taking any herbal medicines for a week or two before your operation.

*Indicates an entry in the A–Z of this book.

# Part 1

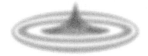

An A–Z of Animal, Mineral
and Vegetable Substances
Used in Medicines

## ACACIA Gum Arabic      *Acacia senegal* (Leguminosae)

The acacia tree grows in North Africa, particularly the Sudan. Gum Arabic is the name given to the air-dried gummy exudate from the stem and branches.

Acacia is used as a suspending and emulsifying agent. It is also used as a tablet binder, and with other ingredients in pastilles, to soothe inflamed tissue, as in irritable bowel, sore throat and bronchial complaints.

See Product Index for EYES.

Also listed among 'other ingredients' of many products.

## ACETIC ACID

*Acetum* is the Latin word for vinegar.

Acetic acid has astringent, antibacterial and antifungal activity, is expectorant and is reported to be spermicidal.

It is used in cough linctuses, for wasp stings and in vaginal preparations.

Acetic acid is a product of fermentation – wine turned to vinegar. Vinegar is a dilute solution of acetic acid which can be used to treat wasp stings, (sodium bicarbonate for bee stings).

See Product Index for COLDS, EARS and PAIN (Topical).

## ACHILLEA – see YARROW

## ACONITE Wolfsbane, Monkshood      *Aconitum napellus* (Ranunculaceae)

NB: Arnica is also called Wolfsbane.

This plant grows in Europe and has violet-blue flowers. The dried roots are used, which contain alkaloids, including aconitine. In the past it was used as an arrow poison.

Aconite is no longer used in conventional medicine as it is very toxic; however it is still used by herbal practitioners in the treatment of heart conditions and as a liniment for treating the pain of neuralgia, rheumatism, lumbago and arthritis, although it should never be applied to wounds or abraded surfaces. Such liniments should be used with care, as sufficient aconitine may be absorbed through the skin to cause serious poisoning.

It is also used in homoeopathic preparations.

See Product Index for COLDS, DIARRHOEA, EARS, FIRST AID, MOUTH, PAIN (Oral), SLEEP and STRESS.

## AESCULUS – see HORSE CHESTNUT

## AGAR Agar agar
*Gelidium cartilagineum* (Gelidiaceae) and other species of seaweed

Indigenous to Japan, many other countries now grow it. The name agar is of Malaysian origin.

This is a gelling agent and is a vegetarian alternative to gelatine (which is made from animal bones). It absorbs moisture quickly, providing bulk and lubrication to the intestinal tract, and so can be used, with other ingredients, for relief of constipation. It is used as an ingredient in emulsions, lotions and suppositories, and as a thickening agent in the food industry. It is widely used as the basis of many culture media for the growth of micro-organisms.

It is normally listed among the 'other ingredients' of products.

## AGNUS CASTUS Chaste Tree
*Vitex agnus castus* (Vibenaceae)

A deciduous, aromatic shrub or small tree found in southern Europe. Its white flowers have long been associated with chastity, particularly in southern Europe.

The dried ripe fruits are used, which contain aucubin and agnuside, which are iridoid glycosides, as well as flavonoids, castin (a bitter), plus fatty and ethereal oils.

Agnus castus acts on the anterior pituitary gland, reducing FSH (follicle-stimulating hormone), and increasing LH (luteinising hormone). Thus it stimulates the production of progesterone in the second half of the menstrual cycle, relative to that of oestrogen.

It also affects prolactin production, increasing or decreasing it, dependent on the dose. Many women who suffer from premenstrual syndrome (PMS) have a heightened sensitivity to prolactin, so a decrease, in conjunction with the increased progesterone helps to reduce PMS, alleviating painful periods, breast pain, water retention and heavy menstrual bleeding. It is used to promote breast milk in nursing mothers and is also useful in teenage acne in both sexes.

It is used in homoeopathic medicine.

It should be avoided by those receiving other forms of sex hormones, for example, HRT and oral contraceptives.

It is sold as a food supplement.

## AGRIMONY Sticklewort    *Agrimonia eupatoria* (Compositae)

This plant grows in Britain, in fields and hedgerows, flowering in July and August. It is named after Eupator, a king of Persia in the 1st century bc, who was famed for his herbal skills.

It contains coumarins, tannins, flavonoids including quercetin* and essential oil.

An ancient remedy for supperating sores and wounds, by cleansing and healing and for chest complaints. It is a mild astringent, diuretic, and a tonic which is now used in herbal medicine for sore throat and laryngitis, indigestion, to promote the flow of gastric juices, and for bed-wetting and incontinence.

See Product Index for HAEMORRHOIDS.

## ALCHEMILLA – see LADY'S MANTLE

## ALEXANDRIAN SENNA – see SENNA

## ALFALFA Lucerne, Purple Medick

*Medicago sativa*
(Leguminosae)

A bushy perennial shrub which originated in Central Asia, which is now widely distributed. The name alfalfa is of Arabic origin, meaning 'best kind of fodder'.

The leaves are used, which contain many active principles including vitamins and minerals: vitamin A* (as Beta-carotene), B6, C, D, E and K, and the minerals* calcium, magnesium, phosphorus and potassium.

Alfalfa is used as an antioxidant, alternative nutrient to promote strong bones and teeth, and to increase weight and vitality. It relieves constipation, is anticholesterol, anti-anaemia and anticoagulant. It is rich in chlorophyll and so stimulates the growth of supportive connective tissue and is useful for collagen diseases, such as arthritis.

Hence its use in both herbal and homoeopathic medicine.

See Product Index for SLEEP. It is also sold as a food supplement.


## ALGINIC ACID and ALGINATES

*Laminaria* species
(Phaeophyceae)

These substances are extracted from algae found in the oceans of the world.

Alginic acid is used in antacid preparations, reacting with the stomach acid to form a raft on the surface of the stomach contents and so preventing the stomach acid from refluxing into the oesophagus.

Alginates are also used as haemostatics, in the form of dressings which, when applied to bleeding surfaces, act as a matrix for coagulation and swell to a gel-like mass; they are used to pack sinuses, fistulas and bleeding tooth sockets, to cover or pack wounds and burns.

They are also used as suspending and thickening agents and also as binding and disintegrating agents in tablet manufacture, and as a demulcent in throat lozenges.

See Product Index for INDIGESTION.

## ALLANTOIN – see COMFREY, CORNSILK, LUNGWORT

Allantoin is astringent and keratolytic and is used in skin preparations for a variety of skin disorders, as well as in haemorrhoidal preparations for its astringent properties.

## ALLSPICE Pimento, Jamaican Pepper
*Pimento dioica*
(Myrtaceae)

An evergreen tree native to the West Indies which flowers from June to August, after which the berries appear and are collected. Allspice is said to combine the flavours of cinnamon, cloves and nutmeg, hence its name.

The unripe fruit contain a volatile oil which comprises a mixture of components including eugenol*, cineole (also found in eucalyptus*) and antioxidants.

The powdered fruit is used as a carminative and aromatic stimulant; it is an ingredient of 'mixed spices', which is used as a condiment; it is also used to aid treatment of flatulence and dyspepsia. The eugenol contained in the volatile oil has antiseptic and local anaesthetic properties.

## ALMOND, SWEET Amygdala dulcis
*Prunus amygdalus*
var. *dulcis* (Rosaceae)

The sweet almond tree came originally from western Asia but is now grown extensively elsewhere. Amygdala is the Latin word for almond.

The fixed oil expressed without the aid of heat from the seeds (nuts) of the almond tree, contains glycerides, mainly oleic acid plus some linoleic, mysteric and palmitic acids.

Almond oil is demulcent and nutritive, being a source of fats and minerals* – iron, calcium, potassium, phosphorus, copper and zinc. It is also emollient and an emulsifier, hence its wide use in aromatherapy as a carrier and massage oil, and in creams and lotions. It can be used to soften ear wax.

See Product Index for EARS and SKIN. It is also sold as a food supplement.

## ALOE VERA                    *Aloe barbadensis* (Liliaceae)

This perennial plant is a native of Africa but grows well anywhere with a warmer climate. Aloe vera gel is present under the outer surface of the leaf, and is obtained by cold-pressing; it contains polysaccharides, anthroquinone glycosides, glycoproteins, sterols, saponins and organic acids.

Widely used in herbal medicine for thousands of years, it is antimicrobial; that is, it has antibiotic, antifungal and antiviral properties as well as being demulcent, astringent, coagulant and analgesic. A rich source of amino acids and vitamins, it helps eliminate toxic minerals from the body and neutralises free radicals created by toxic substances. It is an excellent sunscreen, and can also be used to treat burns and other skin problems, such as acne, eczema, shingles, burns, ulcers, chapped hands, nappy rash and contact dermatitis. It is helpful in treating stretch marks of pregnancy, age lines and liver spots, as well as dry scalp and hair problems. Aloe vera is also used in cosmetics and beauty products – it is claimed that Cleopatra used it for this purpose.

It is sold as a food supplement.

See ALOES for other internal uses of this plant.

## ALOES Barbados Aloes          *Aloe barbadensis* (Liliaceae)
### Cape Aloes                   *Aloe ferox* (Liliaceae)

Aloes are produced by allowing the liquid, from the cut leaves of the aloe plant, to dry solid. This contains anthroquinone glycosides (aloin compounds) and resins.

Aloes is widely used as a laxative, but as it tastes very bitter it has to be given as tablets, and because of a tendency to cause griping, it is usually given in combination with antispasmodics (such as belladonna*) and carminatives. The cleansing effect, due to its action on the digestive tract, makes it useful in the treatment of a number of skin conditions, especially psoriasis, as the process of internal detoxification is considered to be important by herbalists and naturopaths.

The bitter taste is utilised in preparations, such as paints, to discourage nail-biting.

It is also used in homoeopathic medicine.

It should not be taken in pregnancy, nor by nursing mothers, as it is excreted in breast milk.

See Aloe Vera for other uses of this plant. See Product Index for CONSTIPATION.

**ALOIN** – see ALOES

**ALTHAEA** – see MARSHMALLOW

**ALUM** Potash Alum, Aluminium Potassium Sulphate

Occurs naturally in volcanic rocks around the world.

Alum precipitates proteins and is a powerful astringent. It is used solid or in solution as a haemostatic for superficial abrasions, cuts, and as a mouthwash or gargle. When taken internally, large doses are irritant and may be corrosive; adverse effects on muscle and the kidneys have been reported from such misuse.

**ALUMINIUM HYDROXIDE**

Occurs naturally as the mineral Gibbsite, but is now made synthetically.

It is used as a slow-acting antacid in indigestion mixtures. As it tends to cause constipation, it is often given with magnesium hydroxide* or magnesium trisilicate* (antacids that are slightly laxative) to counteract this.

See Product Index for INDIGESTION.

**AMYGDALA DULCIS** – see ALMOND OIL

## ANGELICA, CHINESE Dong Quai *Angelica polymorpha var. sinensis* (Umbelliferrae)

As its name suggests, this plant comes from eastern Asia.

The dried root, which contains a volatile oil, is used for disorders of the female reproductive system. It acts primarily as a tonic, is a mild laxative, sedative and pain-killer, with some antibacterial activity.

Angelica is used in herbal medicine mainly for menstrual, postpartum and menopausal complaints, but also for anaemia, neuralgia and arthritis. It should not be taken by those with clotting disorders, or those taking anticoagulants or awaiting surgery.

## ANGELICA European Archangelica *Angelica archangelica* (Umbellifererae)

This is a common garden plant in Britain and grows wild in Europe and Japan. Angelica means angelic plant, from the medieval Latin, for its reputed power against poison and plague, and also for its sweet scent. In the old (Julian) calender it came into flower around the feast day of Archangel Michael, hence its Latin name.

The dried root and seeds contain a volatile oil, coumarins, flavonoids and sterols.

Angelica is used as a smooth-muscle relaxant, carminative, diuretic, antifungal, antimicrobial, anticatarrhal, expectorant, digestive tonic and antispasmodic for digestive problems, bronchitis, catarrh and influenza, menstrual and obstetric problems.

It is also used in the production of Chartreuse and Benedictine.

It should not be used in pregnancy or diabetes.

See Product Index for COLDS, DIARRHOEA, NAUSEA and STRESS.

## ANISEED *Pimpinella anisum* (Umbelliferae)

This annual herb came originally from Egypt and Asia Minor but is now widely cultivated in warmer climates.

The dried ripe fruit contains a volatile oil (anise oil), plus coumarins and flavonoid glycosides. Anise oil contains anethol, choline* and mucilage.

Aniseed is carminative, expectorant and antispasmodic and hence is used for coughs and bronchitis in cough mixtures and lozenges and also as an aid to digestion. It is also used as a flavouring agent.

See Product Index for COLDS, CONSTIPATION and INDIGESTION.

## ANISE OIL – see ANISEED

## ANTIMONY Stibium

A brittle bluish-white element of metallic appearance.

Antimony is used in anthroposophical ointments for its healing qualities.

See Product Index for HAEMORRHOIDS and SKIN.

## APATITE

This mineral contains a mixture of calcium salts: phosphate, fluoride and chloride.

It is used in homoeopathic medicine.

See Product Index for VITAMINS, MINERALS, TONICS.

## APIS MELLIFERA – see HONEY-BEE

## ARACHIS Peanut, Ground Nut, Earth Nut
*Arachis hypogaea*
(Leguminosae)

The plant is native to tropical Africa, and is now cultivated widely.

The fixed oil is expressed from the nuts; it contains glycerides, chiefly oleic and linoleic acids, as well as bioflavonoids, tannins and vitamins* B1, B2, B3 and E.

It is used both internally – emulsions containing arachis oil are used in nutrition; and externally as an emollient, in creams, lotions, soaps, enemas and for softening ear wax.

Unrefined arachis oil should not be used in infancy to prevent sensitisation. Most manufacturers now use refined oil, from which the proteins that cause the allergic reaction in susceptible people have been removed.

Those allergic to peanuts should avoid any preparations containing arachis oil and should note the alternative names given above which are also sometimes used by manufacturers. People with a nut allergy, who are at risk of anaphylaxis, should always carry an Epipen, so that they can immediately inject adrenaline, to prevent anaphylactic shock, should they come into contact with nuts. Such an injection is only first aid though; the patient must go to hospital immediately for further treatment.

See Product Index for EARS, FEET and SKIN.

## ARECA – see BETEL NUTS

## ARNICA Leopard's Bane, Wolfsbane — *Arnica montana* (Compositae)

NB: Aconite is also called Wolfsbane.

The plant is native to Europe, apart from Britain, and is also cultivated in north India.

The name is said to be derived from the Greek, meaning lambskin, a reference to the texture of its leaves.

The dried flower-heads contain flavonoids, sesquiterpene lactones, volatile oil (which contains thymol*), mucilage, polysaccharides, resins, bitters and tannins. Arnica is aromatic, diuretic, stimulant and vulnerary, as well as being insecticidal and acting as a counterirritant. It is used to prepare tinctures, creams and lotions for treating bruises and sprains, where the skin is unbroken and not too tender, but arnica may cause dermatitis when applied to the skin of sensitive persons.

It is widely used in herbal and homoeopathic preparations.

See Product Index for EYES, FIRST AID, MOUTH, PAIN (Oral), PAIN (Topical) and SKIN.

## ARROWROOT — *Maranta arundinacea* (Marantaceae)

A herbaceous plant, native to Tropical America and the West Indies taking its name from its use as an antidote to arrow poison.

Arrowroot, a white odourless, tasteless powder which is the starch granules of the rhizomes. It has the general properties of starch, being nutritive and demulcent.

It is used as a gruel in the treatment of diarrhoea: one tablespoon to one pint of boiling water produces a suitable demulcent mucilage.

## ARTICHOKE Globe Artichoke
*Cynara scolymus*
(Compositae)

A perennial plant native to the Mediterranean region and North Africa.

The leaves and blossom contain cynarin, cynaropicrin and phenolic acids. Cynarin protects and enhances liver function, cynaropicrin stimulates liver function and the phenolic acids reduce blood cholesterol and lipid levels.

Thus artichoke relieves dyspepsia, reduces cholesterol, stimulates the flow of bile and is anti-emetic and antioxidant, and is used for digestive, liver and gall bladder problems, also it reduces the level of fats in the blood, stimulates the metabolism, reduces fluid retention and detoxifies. It may also benefit those who suffer from irritable bowel syndrome.

See Product Index for INDIGESTION. It is also sold as a food supplement.

## ASAFETIDA Devil's Dung     *Ferula asafoetida* (Umbelliferae)

A perennial plant that grows widely from the Mediterranean to central Asia. The name is derived from Persian *aza*, meaning mastic, and Latin *fetida*, meaning stinking.

An oleo-gum-resin is obtained from the living rhizome and root, which has a garlic-like odour and a bitter, acrid taste.

Asefetida is a powerful expectorant, carminative, antispasmodic, and is also anti-inflammatory; and although it has no pain-killing activity, it has been shown to produce improvement in arthritis and rheumatism. It is also helpful for stress and nerves. It is used in cooking and is an ingredient of certain foods, including Lea & Perrins Worcestershire sauce.

See Product Index for SLEEP.

**ASCORBIC ACID** – see VITAMIN C

**ATROPINE** – see BELLADONNA, also present in HENBANE and THORNAPPLE

## ATTAPULGITE

This is a type of mineral detergent clay which consists of a purified native aluminium magnesium silicate.

Activated attapulgite is highly absorbent and adsorbent and is used as a suspending and emulsifying agent; suspensions containing it are thixotropic.

It is used in a wide range of products including fertilisers, pesticides and pharmaceuticals, such as anti-diarrhoeal preparations.

See Product Index for DIARRHOEA.

**AVENA** – see OAT

**BALM OF GILEAD** – see POPLAR BUDS

**BARBADOS ALOES** – see ALOES

**BARBERRY** Berberis          *Berberis vulgaris* (Berberidaceae)

This common bush grows in Britain and Europe. The bark from the stems and roots, also the roots and berries, contain alkaloids including berberine, as well as tannins and resin.

Barberry is antipyretic, anti-inflammatory, antiseptic and antibacterial, hypotensive, anti-emetic, sedative and a uterine stimulant; because berberine stimulates the secretion of bile and bilirubin it is used for sluggish liver, gallstones, digestive, skin and bladder disorders.

It should not be used in pregnancy.

**BARLEY**          *Hordeum distichon* (Gramineae)

A grass which is cultivated throughout the world.

An almost perfect food, which is high in fibre, lysine (an essential amino-acid), and also the minerals* calcium, iron (good for anaemia), magnesium and potassium.

Barley is anticholesterol, demulcent, nutritive and, taken as barley water, is still used in kidney, intestinal and bowel disorders, such as constipation. See also Malt Extract*.

**BAY, LAUREL**          *Laurus nobilis* (Lauraceae)

This large bush or tree is a native of the Mediterranean and is widely cultivated.

The leaves contain a volatile oil that contains mainly cineole.

The oil from laurel leaves and stems or from the berries is antiseptic, antifungal and antidandruff. It is carminative, acting as a gastric tonic and is used in urinary infections, as it is also diuretic.

## BAY, MYRCIA          *Pimenta acris* (Myrtaceae)

This tree grows in the West Indies.

The oil is used in the preparation of bay rum (Rhum), which is used as a hair lotion and as an astringent, applied to the face after shaving.

See Product Index for HAIR.


## BAYBERRY Wax Myrtle          *Myrica cerifera* (Myricaceae)

An evergreen shrub or small tree native to North America, now widely cultivated in Europe and the British Isles. The bark from the root contains triterpenes, flavonoids, tannins, phenols, resins and gums.

Bayberry is used as a circulatory stimulant, tonic and astringent and is diaphoretic and anticoagulant; it is also antimicrobial and spermicidal, and is used for congestive catarrhal conditions, colitis, irritable bowel syndrome and diarrhoea.

See Product Index for COLDS.


## BEARBERRY Uva Ursi     *Arctostaphylos uva-ursi* (Ericaceae)

A small evergreen shrub which grows in Britain, Europe and North America. The dried leaves contain hydroquinones, iridoids, flavonoids, phenolic compounds and tannins.

Bearberry is diuretic, astringent, antimicrobial and haemostatic; it has been used in the treatment of urethritis, pyelitis and cystitis. It is also used in homoeopathic medicine.

It should not be used in pregnancy, or whilst breast-feeding, or in kidney disorders.

See Product Index for PAIN (Oral), STRESS and URINARY TRACT.

It is also sold as a food supplement. Long-term use is not recommended.


## BEESWAX

Beeswax is produced by the honey-bee* to build the honeycomb. The wax is obtained by melting the honeycomb with hot water and removing any foreign matter.

It is used as an ingredient in ointments and sometimes suppositories.

Beeswax is also used to make furniture polishes.

See Product Index for FEET and SKIN; also listed in 'other ingredients' of many products.

## BELLADONNA Deadly Nightshade      *Atropa belladonna*
(Solanaceae)

A perennial plant that grows wild in Britain and parts of Europe, which is collected when in flower.

The dried leaves and flowering tops contain alkaloids, including atropine, hyoscyamine (which is an isomer of atropine), and some hyoscine.

The root also contains these alkaloids but is used mainly for external preparations, such as liniments and plasters and as counterirritants to relieve pain.

Belladonna herb is used in preparations for the treatment of intestinal and biliary colic, due to its antispasmodic action on smooth muscle, and has been used in conjunction with vegetable laxatives to prevent griping.

Atropine is used in eye-drops for treating various eye disorders by dilating the pupil. Centuries ago it was used by young ladies to make them look more alluring, which is how the plant got the name belladonna (beautiful lady).

It is widely used in homoeopathic medicine.

It should not be used in pregnancy, or by men with an enlarged prostate gland.

See Product Index for INDIGESTION and also for COLDS, DIARRHOEA, EARS, FIRST AID, NAUSEA & TRAVEL SICKNESS, PAIN (Oral) and SKIN.

## BENTONITE

This is native colloidal aluminium silicate, a sort of clay. It is named after Fort Benton, Montana, USA, where it was first found.

It swells in water and so is used for suspending powders in aqueous solutions, such as Calamine Lotion, and for making gels as well as for ointment and cream bases.

It has been used as a bulk laxative and also as an oral adsorbent, for example in the treatment of paraquat poisoning.

See Product Index for FIRST AID.

## BENZOIC ACID

It is present in some plants; and being antibacterial and antifungal is used to treat fungal infections of the skin. It is also used in mouthwashes and as a food preservative.

See Product Index for COLDS, FEET and SKIN.

### BENZOIN Gum Benzoin    *Styrax benzoin* (Styracaceae)

This gum tree grows in Sumatra and Java.

Benzoin is a balsamic resin or gum collected from the incised stem, which contains balsamic acids, present as the esters of benzoic and cinnamic acids.

It is astringent, carminative and expectorant, hence its use as an ingredient of inhalations to treat catarrh. It also has antiseptic and protective properties and so is used in topical preparations. Friar's Balsam is the common name for Benzoin Compound Tincture.

See Product Index for COLDS, HAEMORRHOIDS and SKIN.

### BERGAMOT    *Citrus bergamia* (Rutaceae)

The bergamot orange tree is an evergreen which is native to South-East Asia and the Pacific islands. The oil, which is obtained by expression from the fresh peel of the fruit, is aromatic, antiseptic, carminative and antispasmodic. Bergamot oil is chiefly used in perfumery and suntan preparations, as well as diluted in aromatherapy.

### BETA-CAROTENE – see VITAMIN A

### BETEL    *Areca catechu* (Palmae)

This evergreen palm grows in India, Malaysia, Australia and the Solomon Islands.

The dried ripe fruits (betel nuts) contain alkaloids, chiefly arecoline, tannins and fixed oil. The nuts are astringent and stimulant and are chewed in Asia, staining red the lips, teeth and excrement. It acts as an anthelmintic to expel tapeworms.

## BILBERRY Blueberry, Huckleberry — *Vaccinium myrtillus* (Vacciniaceae)

A deciduous shrub which grows mainly on moorland, heaths and on other acid soils in the UK, Europe and North America.

The ripe fruit (berries) contain anthocyanosides (a type of flavonoid), vitamin C* and plant acids such as citric acid* and malic acid.

The anthocyanosides, which are antioxidants, are able to bind to the retina of the eye, thus increasing the rate of regeneration of the visual pigments produced in the retina; hence it is used in herbal medicine for eye strain and to improve vision. Bilberry can also prevent destruction of collagen and reduce blood sugar levels.

Bilberry is astringent, diuretic and refrigerant (relieves thirst and gives a feeling of coolness), and is used in herbal medicine to treat diarrhoea, ophthalmic and circulatory disorders; however, it is mainly used as a food.

It is also used in homoeopathic medicine and is sold as a food supplement.

## BIOTIN – see VITAMINS

## BIRCH European Birch, Silver Birch — *Betula alba* (Betulacea)

The silver birch is a common tree in the woodlands of Britain and Europe.

The bark and leaves are used; they contain flavonoids, saponins and salicylates which have an aspirin-like effect, being analgesic and anti-inflammatory.

The young leaves have a diuretic effect. Birch is also bitter and astringent and is used in herbal medicine for rheumatism and gout, as a gargle for sore mouths and for cellulitis.

See Product Index for PAIN (Oral and Topical) and TONICS.

## BITTERSWEET Woody Nightshade    *Solanum dulcamara*
(Solanaceae)

This plant, which has purple and yellow flowers, grows wild in Britain, Europe, Asia and North Africa.

The twigs and root bark contain dulcamarin, a saponin glycoside.

An astringent herb with a bitter then sweet taste, hence its name. It lowers fever and has expectorant, diuretic, sedative, narcotic, stimulant and antirheumatic effects. It is used for chronic bronchitis, for gout and rheumatism, and externally for warts and ulcers as well as eczema.

It should not be used in pregnancy or while breast-feeding.

It should be used with care as all parts, especially the leaves and unripe berries, are poisonous if eaten.

See Product Index for INDIGESTION and SKIN.


## BLACK BRYONY – see BRYONY, BLACK


## BLACK COHOSH Black Snakeroot    *Cimifuga racemosa*
(Ranunculaceae)

A hardy perennial which grows in temperate regions of North America. Black cohosh is used by the American Indians for female problems – they call it squaw root.

The root and rhizome contain triterpene glycosides, isoflavones and salicylic acid.

Black cohosh, an immune stimulant which is astringent, diuretic, expectorant, hypotensive and anti-obese, is also sedative, antispasmodic, antiarthritic, antirheumatic and antigout due to the salicylic acid content which has an anti-inflammatory and analgesic aspirin-like effect. It is also useful for sciatica and low back pain, neuralgia and aches caused by strenuous exercise. It acts powerfully on the female reproductive system, for painful periods and menopausal symptoms, and is also useful for painful breasts and migraine of hormonal origin.

In homoeopathic medicine it is known as Actaea racemosa or Actaea rac.

Black cohosh should not be taken by those allergic to aspirin.

It should not be taken in pregnancy or whilst breast-feeding,

It should not be taken by those who have, or have had in the past, an oestrogen-dependent (that is, oestrogen-receptor-positive) tumour such as breast, endometrial, cervical or ovarian cancer, as evidence of safety is not yet proven.

See Product Index for COLDS and PAIN (Oral). It is also sold as a food supplement.


## BLACK HAW American Sloe — *Vibernum prunifolium* (Caprifoliaceae)

A deciduous shrub with brilliant autumn colour, from Eastern and central USA.

The stem and root bark are used, which contain coumarins (including scopoletin), salicin, vibernin, plant acids, volatile oil and tannin.

Black haw is a uterine tonic, and is sedative, nervine, hypotensive, anti-asthmatic, antispasmodic, diuretic and antidiarrhoeal. The uterine sedative effects are due to the scopoletin it contains.

It is used to prevent miscarriage in the last few weeks of pregnancy, for dysmenorrhoea, and after childbirth to reduce pain and bleeding, (due to the salicin content). It is also used to treat flooding which can occur in the menopause.

See Product Index for PAIN (Oral) and ADDENDA for WOMEN only.


## BLACK ROOT Culver's Physic — *Veronicastrum virginicum* (Scrophulariaceae)

A perennial from eastern North America, used by the Indians and first tried by a settler, Dr Culver; it was then introduced in Europe in 1714.

The dried root and rhizome contain saponins and volatile oil.

Black root is antiseptic, diaphoretic, stomachic, tonic, antispasmodic and laxative without griping. It stimulates the liver and gall bladder and is used for indigestion associated with liver complaints, and for constipation.

See Product Index for INDIGESTION.

**BLACK SAMPSON** – see ECHINACEA

**BLACK SNAKEROOT** – see BLACK COHOSH

**BLACK TANG** – see BLADDERWRACK

**BLACKBERRY** Bramble         *Rubus villosus* **(Rosaceae)**

A prickly low-growing plant found in Britain and Europe.

The leaves and root bark are used. They contain tannin, flavonoid glycosides, malic acid and pectin.

Blackberry is a powerful astringent and haemostatic. It is a diaphoretic febrifuge, which is refrigerant and diuretic and is used as a gargle for sore throats and for mouth ulcers and bleeding gums. It has also been used by herbal practitioners, for diarrhoea and dysentery and bleeding from the colon and rectum.

See Product Index for DIARRHOEA.

**BLACKCURRANT**         *Ribes nigrum* **(Grossulariaceae)**

A deciduous shrub which grows in northern temperate regions.

The fresh ripe fruit are a rich source of vitamin C*. The leaves contain flavonoids, glycosides, tannins and essential oil. The seeds are rich in gamolenic acid*.

Blackcurrant is astringent, tonic and anti-inflammatory; it is also antibacterial and is used for colds, mouth and throat infections as well as sore throats.

See Product Index for COLDS.

**BLACKTHORN** Sloe         *Prunus spinosa* **(Rosaceae)**

A deciduous tree found in Britain and Europe.

The flowers contain flavonoids and cyanogenic glycosides. In addition to these, the fruits contain mainly tannins, pectin*, organic acids and vitamin C*.

It is diuretic, anti-inflammatory and astringent.

The flowers are used as a diuretic, mild laxative and to strengthen the walls of blood capillaries, whilst the fruits are used in digestive disorders. They are also used as a mouthwash or gargle for inflammation of the mouth and throat.

The fresh fruits are used in making home-made wine and sloe gin.

See Product Index for COLDS and TONICS.

## BLADDERWRACK Kelpware, Seawrack, Black Tang *Fucus vesiculosis* (Fucaceae)

This is a seaweed which is commonly found in colder waters, such as around Britain.

The dried plant contains a gelatinous substance (algin), and minerals* sodium, manganese, sulphur, silicon, zinc, copper* and some iodine*, which is the reason people take it when trying to lose weight. Iodine is essential for the correct functioning of the thyroid gland which governs the body's metabolic rate. It is alternative and hence is beneficial for the male and female reproductive organs, as well as the liver, gall bladder and pancreas. It militates against the onset of rheumatism and arthritis, and is a source of vitamin K* for the prevention of strokes.

It is used in herbal and homoeopathic medicine.

Bladderwrack should not be taken by those with high blood pressure, kidney disorders or thyroid conditions, without first consulting the doctor and should not be used in pregnancy.

See Product Index for PAIN (Oral), SLIMMING and URINARY TRACT.

## BLAZING STAR – see FALSE UNICORN ROOT

## BLESSED THISTLE – see HOLY THISTLE

## BLUE FLAG Iris Versicolor *Iris versicolor* (Iridaceae)

This iris is commonly grown in British gardens, and grows wild in parts of North America.

The dried rhizome and root contain volatile oil, a glycoside (iridin), gum, resin and sterols.

Blue flag is antibiotic, anti-inflammatory, astringent, diuretic, laxative, stimulant and anti-obese. A powerful alternative for passive, sluggish conditions involving the liver, gall bladder, lymphatics and veins. It promotes the secretions of the pancreas, intestines and salivary glands.

It is used in herbal and homoeopathic medicine.

See Product Index for COLDS and SKIN. It is also sold as a food supplement.

## BLUE GUM – see EUCALYPTUS

## BOGBEAN – see BUCKBEAN

## BOLDO                             *Peumus boldus* (Monimiaceae)

An evergreen shrub or small tree found only in Chile. The dried leaves contain the alkaloid boldine, the glycoside boldoglucin and some volatile oil.

Boldo is sedative, tonic and antigout and is used in herbal medicine as a diuretic and urinary antiseptic, hence its use for fluid retention, cystitis and also a mild laxative. It is anti-obese and anti-inflammatory; and as it acts on the gall bladder, it is used for gallstones and liver complaints.

See Product Index for SLIMMING. It is also sold as a food supplement.

## BONESET Feverwort              *Eupatorium perfoliatum*
                                              (Compositae)

A perennial herb which grows in North America. The whole plant is used, which contains immunostimulatory polysaccharides, lactones, flavonoids, sterols and a little volatile oil.

Boneset is a bitter, astringent herb which is diaphoretic, expectorant, laxative, stimulant and tonic, antiviral and antipruritic, and stimulates the immune system and reduces fever and pain in bones, hence its name. Large doses can be emetic.

It is used for colds, catarrh, influenza, bronchitis and for some skin diseases.

See Product Index for COLDS.

## BORACIC ACID = BORIC ACID

Both names are used for the same substance which has weak bacteriostatic and fungistatic properties but has been superceded by more effective and less toxic disinfectants. It is no longer used internally, but is still used as a buffer in eye-drops.

If it is used to bathe raw or weeping surfaces sufficient can be absorbed to cause poisoning, so it is no longer used, as other, safer agents are available.

## BORAGE – see GAMOLENIC ACID

## BORAX Sodium Borate

It occurs naturally in sedimentary borate deposits.

Borax is not used internally but is used as an emulsifying agent with beeswax in cold creams.

It is a mild alkali and so can be used to remove stains from fabrics.

## BORIC ACID – see BORACIC ACID

## BRAN

The fibrous outer layers of cereal grains, usually wheat. Bran contains celluloses, polysaccharides, protein, fat and minerals. It absorbs nine times its own weight of water and therefore, when added to the diet, forms easily passed, soft, moist stools, so regulating bowel function; thus it may be of use in both constipation and diaorrhea. In the past bran has been recommended to patients with irritable bowel syndrome, however recent trials have shown that it causes as many problems as it solves. It is present in many breakfast cereals.

## BREWER'S YEAST – see YEAST

## BROMELAIN – see PINEAPPLE

## BRYONY, BLACK      *Tamus communis* (Dioscoeaceae)

This plant grows in hedgerows in Britain.

The root contains glycosides.

Black bryony is used by herbal practitioners as a diuretic and also externally as a rubefacient for gout and rheumatism.

See Product Index for SKIN.

## BRYONY, WHITE      *Bryonia dioica* (Cucurbitacea)

This plant grows in England and parts of central and southern Europe.

The root of the plant is used in homoeopathic medicine for respiratory infections and inflammatory disorders.

See Product Index for COLDS, CONSTIPATION, INDIGESTION and PAIN (Oral).

## BUCHU      *Barosma betulina* (Rutaceae)

This plant comes from South Africa and has been classed as an official medicine in Britain for over 150 years.

The dried leaves contain a volatile oil, flavonoids, B vitamins*, tannin and mucilage.

Buchu is a weak diuretic, and is used for fluid retention, and also as a urinary antiseptic for cystitis. It is antimicrobial, diaphoretic and stimulant.

It is used in homoeopathic medicine.

See Product Index for PAIN (Oral), SKIN and URINARY.

It is also sold as a food supplement.

## BUCKBEAN Bogbean      *Menyanthes trifoliata* (Menyanthaceae)

An aquatic or creeping perennial which grows in marshy ground in Britain and Europe.

The dried leaves are used, to produce a bitter, which contains iridoid glycosides, alkaloids, flavonoids and coumarins.

Buckbean is used in herbal medicine as an ingredient in tonics as it is a bitter hepatic; it is also used as a diuretic, febrifuge, anti-inflammatory and antirheumatic. It is laxative in large doses.

It is also used in homoeopathic medicine

See Product Index for PAIN (Oral).

## BUCKTHORN Alder Buckthorn

*Frangula alnus* (Rhamnaceae)

A small tree which grows in Britain, Europe and in America.

The dried, ripe fruit are used; also the inner bark is used, but only after two years of drying, as the fresh bark causes griping.

Buckthorn contains anthraquinone glycosides and acts as a bitter, a diuretic, and a stimulating laxative in chronic spastic constipation.

It is not recommended for use in pregnancy, while breast-feeding or for children.

See Product Index for CONSTIPATION.

## BURDOCK

*Arctium lappa* (Compositae)

It grows wild in Europe, parts of Asia and in North America.

The dried stems, root and seeds are used. They contain amino acids, phenolic acids and fatty acids, sesquiterpenes, inulin, tannin and mucilage. A source of iron, sulphur and the B vitamins*.

This herb is a bitter, alternative, antihistamine, diaphoretic, aphrodisiac, diuretic, laxative which also lowers blood sugar. The root is antibiotic, antifungal, antiviral, antigout and anti-inflammatory.

It is used internally to treat skin diseases and inflammatory conditions due to toxicity, such as eczema, psoriasis, boils, sores, rheumatism and gout.

See Product Index for COLDS, INDIGESTION, PAIN (Oral), SKIN and URINARY TRACT.

It is also sold as a food supplement.

## BUTTERBUR Bog Rhubarb

*Petasites lybridus*
(Compositae)

This plant grows in boggy places throughout Europe.

The herb contains pyrrolizidine alkaloids, sesquiterpene lactones, volatile oil, pectin and mucilage. The root contains inulin.

Butterbur is tonic, stimulant, expectorant, anti-infective, antispasmodic, anti-inflammatory, analgesic and diuretic and so is used for chest problems, such as bronchitis, asthma and whooping cough. It is also used for colds, fevers, headache, migraine, hay fever and urinary complaints.

The pyrrolizidine alkaloids are toxic to the liver, hence this herb should not be used in excessive doses and should not be used in pregnancy or while breast-feeding. Some manufacturers now remove them during preparation of their products.

It is sold as a food supplement.

## BUTTERFLY WEED – see PLEURISY ROOT

## BUTTERNUT White Walnut

*Juglans cinerea*
(Juglandaceae)

This tree grows in the USA.

The root bark and leaves are used, which contain naphthaquinones, fixed and essential oils and tannins.

Butternut acts on the liver and bowel, and also as a blood tonic and is used for chronic constipation associated with liver disease, to increase the flow of bile and its release from the gall bladder. It is also anthelmintic.

See Product Index for SLIMMING.

## CADE                    *Juniperus oxycedrus* (Cupressaceae)

A coniferous tree found in the northern hemisphere.

Cade oil is obtained by destructive distillation of the branches and wood of the tree and is antipruritic and slightly antiseptic and is used as an ingredient in ointments and shampoos in the treatment of psoriasis. The ointment is also used to treat eczema. It has been used in medicated soaps and shampoos.

See Product Index for HAIR and SKIN.

## CAFFEINE

This alkaloid is present in tea*, cocoa*, coffee*, guarana*, kola* and maté*.

It acts as a central-nervous-system stimulant and diuretic.

Caffeine is used as an ingredient in many pain-killers because it increases the analgesic effects of paracetamol and aspirin and produces a feeling of wellbeing. Kola is used in drinks, some of which can contain as much as 20 mg of caffeine in 100 ml of liquid.

Women who are pregnant, or hoping to become so, should reduce their daily caffeine intake to below 300 mg (about 4 cups per day), as it has been found that excessive consumption can cause miscarriage or low birth weight of the baby. Decaffeinated coffee and tea are available.

See Product Index for COLDS and VITAMINS, MINERALS and TONICS.

## CAJUPUT Cajeput,              *Melaleuca leucadendron*
##        Swamp Tea Tree                   (Myrtaceae)

A large evergreen tree native to the wetland areas of northern Australia, southern New Guinea and the Molucca Islands. Cajuput is Malaysian for white tree.

Cajuput oil is obtained by distillation of the fresh leaves and twigs; it contains cineole (also found in eucalyptus*). The oil is antiseptic, calminative, antispasmodic and expectorant, and externally is counterirritant and rubefacient; it is also insect repellent.

Cajuput oil is used in ointments and lotions for painful, stiff joints, bruises, sprains and neuralgia; also for relief of respiratory conditions in inhalants.

See Product Index for COLDS, EARS and PAIN (Topical).

## CALAMINE

A mineral, smithsonite, which is a basic zinc carbonate coloured with iron oxide.

Calamine has a mild astringent and antipruritic action on the skin and is used in dusting powders, creams, oinments and lotions for a variety of skin conditions.

See Product Index for FIRST AID.

## CALAMUS – see SWEET FLAG

## CALCIFEROL – see VITAMIN D

## CALCIUM – see CALCIUM CARBONATE and MINERALS

## CALCIUM CARBONATE Chalk

Chalk is a sedimentary deposit formed from the shells of Foraminifera.

Calcium carbonate is widely used in indigestion remedies as an antacid, releasing carbon dioxide on contact with the stomach acid, which may cause flatulence. Excessive use may cause constipation, so it is also sometimes used to treat diarrhoea. It is used as a calcium supplement in deficiency states and as an adjunct in the treatment of osteoporosis.

It is also used as a polishing agent in tooth powders.

See Product Index for COLDS, DIARRHOEA, INDIGESTION, SKIN, STRESS, and VITAMINS, MINERALS and TONICS.

## CALCIUM SULPHATE Gypsum, Plaster of Paris

Gypsum is used as an inert excipient in tablet manufacture.

Plaster of Paris, which is dried calcium sulphate, is mixed with water and then used with bandages to make casts for broken bones.

## CALENDULA – see MARIGOLD

## CALUMBA                    *Jateorhiza palmata* (Menispermaceae)

It grows in east Africa and Madagascar and is now cultivated in Europe.

The dried root contains a bitter which has been used as a tincture for dyspepsia and as a flavouring agent in the formulation of liqueurs. It also contains a volatile oil containing thymol* and alkaloids, but no tannin.

Calumba is a bitter, carminative febrifuge, which acts mainly as a tonic to the digestive system; it is also a uterine stimulant, and is antifungal, sedative and lowers blood pressure, and is used mainly for digestive and menstrual complaints.

It should not be used in pregnancy.

See Product Index for INDIGESTION.

## CAMPHOR                    *Cinnamomum camphora* (Lauraceae)

An evergreen tree found in forests from tropical Asia to Japan.

Camphor is obtained by distillation from the wood.

It is aromatic, diaphoretic, antiseptic, antimicrobial and antispasmodic. Applied externally, camphor acts as a rubefacient and mild analgesic, and is widely used in liniments as a counterirritant for fibrositis, neuralgia and similar conditions. It is also an ingredient of inhaled nasal decongestants.

Camphorated oil is no longer used because of its toxicity: it is absorbed through the skin and can cause camphor-poisoning. Camphor crosses the placenta and so should not be used in pregnancy, and also not by epileptics as it can induce fits. It should not be applied to the nostrils of infants, as this may cause immediate collapse.

See Product Index for COLDS, EARS, FEET and PAIN (Topical).

**CANTHARIS** – see SPANISH FLY

**CAPE ALOES** – see ALOES

## CAPSICUM Red Pepper, Cayenne, Chillies

*Capsicum annum var. minimum*
(Solanaceae)

This pepper grows in tropical America and Africa.

The dried ripe pods which, when powdered, are called cayenne pepper, contain capsaicin, carotenoids and steroidal saponins. Capsicum oleoresin (also called capsicin) is an alcoholic extract containing up to 0.5% capsaicin, the active ingredient of capsicum.

Capsicum is antibiotic and antimicrobial, diaphoretic, anticatarrhal, an anti-emetic, haemostatic, cardiac tonic. It has a carminative and stimulant action, opening up every tissue of the body to an increased flow of blood, and is also antispasmodic for relief of pain. Whilst it is mainly used externally as a counterirritant in lumbago, neuralgia and rheumatism, it is also used for painful skin conditions. Contact with the eyes and broken skin should be avoided. Wash hands after use. It is also used in homoeopathic medicine.

See Product Index for COLDS, INDIGESTION, PAIN (Topical) and SKIN.

## CARAWAY *Carum carvi* (Umbelliferae)

The plant is native to Europe, Asia and North Africa. The Arabic word for the seed, *karawya*, gives us the present name.

The dried ripe fruits contain a volatile oil and flavonoids.

Caraway is antimicrobial, carminative, stomachic, antispasmodic, stimulant and expectorant, and is used as an aromatic carminative for the flatulent colic of babies.

It is also used as a flavouring agent and the seeds are used in cookery.

See Product Index for CONSTIPATION and INDIGESTION.

## CARDAMOM   *Elettaria cardamomum var. miniscula*
(Zingiberaceae)

A perennial plant from the Indian rainforests.

Only the seeds are used, and are removed from the fruit only when needed, as the seeds should not be stored after removal from the fruit.

The seeds contain a volatile oil which is used as an aromatic, carminative, stomachic and stimulant, and also has antispasmodic activity and is so used for digestive problems.

See Product Index for INDIGESTION.

## CAROB BEAN St John's Bread   *Ceratonia siliqua*
(Leguminosae)

This plant is native to south-east Europe and western Asia, now cultivated elsewhere.

The fruit is a woody pod containing a sweet yellow pulp that is made into flour.

The pulp is nutritive and diuretic, containing sugars, fats, starch, proteins and amino acids and is used as a thickener and stabilising agent in the food industry.

It is sold as a food supplement.

## CARRAGEEN – see IRISH MOSS

## CASCARA Cascara Sagrada, Sacred Bark   *Rhamnus purshiana*
(Rhamnaceae)

A thorny tree or shrub native to the Pacific coast of North America.

The dried bark is collected in the spring and early summer, at least a year before it is used. It contains anthroquinone glycosides.

Cascara is a non-habit-forming stimulant laxative and stool softener, best taken at night for results the next morning. It is also used for dyspepsia and in the treatment of piles.

See Product Index for CONSTIPATION, HAEMORRHOIDS and SKIN.

## CASTOR

*Ricinus communis* (Euphorbiaceae)

The castor bean, though native to India, is grown throughout the world.

The fixed oil, expressed from the seeds without the aid of heat, contains triglycerides of ricinoleic acid. The seeds contain a poisonous protein (ricin) which is left behind when the oil is expressed.

When taken by mouth, particularly in large doses, castor oil may produce nausea, vomiting, colic and severe purgation. It should be taken with caution during pregnancy and menstruation.

Castor oil is used externally for its emollient effect, when applied to warts, corns, bunions, psoriasis and eczema and other skin disorders. It is also antifungal.

See Product Index for CONSTIPATION.

## CATECHU

*Uncaria gambier* (Rubiaceae)

This plant comes from south-east Asia.

A dried aqueous extract of the leaves and young shoots, containing flavonoids, tannins and indole alkaloids.

Catechu is astringent, antiseptic and antibacterial and is used for irritable bowel, colitis, catarrh, mouth ulcers and sore throats.

See Product Index for DIARRHOEA.

## CAT'S CLAW

*Uncaria tomentosa* (Malphigiacaea)

This large woody vine comes from the South American rainforests. It gets its name from the hook-like thorns that grow along its stems, *uncus* is Latin for hook.

It is a powerful immune stimulant and anti-inflammatory, and is used for rheumatic and arthritic conditions as well as other conditions where the immune system is compromised, such as glandular fever and ME (myalgic encephalomyelitis). The anti-inflammatory effect gives relief of joint pain and discomfort and also exerts a cleansing and healing effect on the digestive system.

It is sold as a food supplement.

**CAYENNE** – see CAPSICUM

## CELANDINE, GREATER   *Chelidonium majus* (Papaveraceae)

A common plant throughout Europe. Do not confuse with lesser celandine (pilewort*).

The celandine is so named because it flowers at the time of the arrival of the swallows in the spring – celandine being derived from the Greek word for swallow.

This herb contains alkaloids, including berberine and chelidonine which have antiviral activity, also choline*, histamine, saponins, carotene and vitamin C*.

Celandine is an alternative and diuretic herb which has been used in the treatment of eczema and jaundice. The fresh juice can be used as a treament for warts and corns, but not on the face and not by diabetics. It is also antispasmodic, antifungal and antibacterial.

It is used in herbal medicine for eye infections, warts, liver and gall bladder problems and skin disorders.

See Product Index for INDIGESTION.

## CELANDINE, LESSER – see PILEWORT

## CELERY                    *Apium graveolens* (Umbelliferae)

This plant is cultivated widely; the wild plant grows in marshy places.

The dried, ripe fruits contain a volatile oil, which is used as an antispasmodic. Celery is also rich in minerals*, such as iron, phosphorus, potassium and sodium.

Celery is a carminative and digestive tonic, and is hypotensive, anti-inflammatory, antigout and antirheumatic, as well as a diuretic and urinary antiseptic. It is aromatic, stimulant, aphrodisiac, nervine and antidepressant. Celery can also be taken to increase the milk flow in nursing mothers, but should not be taken in pregnancy.

See Product Index for PAIN (Topical) and URINARY TRACT.

It is also sold as a food supplement.

## CENTAURY Feverwort
*Centaurium erythraea*
(Gentianaceae)

This plant is native to Europe, including the British Isles, Western Asia and North Africa. The medicinal properties of this plant were said to have been discovered by the centaur, Chiron, in Greek mythology, hence its Latin name.

The herb contains glycosides, alkaloids, phenolic acids and sterols.

Centaury is bitter, aromatic, carminative, stomachic and tonic, and is used in herbal medicine for digestive disorders, dyspepsia, liver and gall bladder complaints and to stimulate the appetite.

See Product Index for CONSTIPATION.


## CETRARIA ISLANDICA – see ICELAND MOSS


## CHALK – see CALCIUM CARBONATE


## CHAMOMILE Roman Chamomile
*Anthemis nobilis*
(Compositae)

NB: for German Chamomile – see MATRICARIA

This plant is widely cultivated in Europe. The flowers have an apple-like scent from which chamomile gets its name. It means earth-apple in Greek. Chamomile is also called the plant's physician because any plant growing near it will thrive.

The dried flower-heads contain flavonoids and a volatile oil.

Chamomile has been used as an aromatic bitter, although large doses are emetic; Chamomile tea is a remedy for indigestion, for its carminative, anti-inflammatory and antispasmodic effects. Chamomile is a decongestant, analgesic, a mild tranquilliser and sedative, and has antidepressant and anticonvulsant properties. Ointments containing the extract, which is soothing and antiseptic, are used for cracked nipples and nappy rash. It is also an ingredient of shampoos and hair rinses for blonde hair.

It is used in homoeopathic medicine and the essential oil is used in aromatherapy.

Chamomile should not be taken orally in pregnancy.

See Product Index for EARS, INDIGESTION, PAIN (Oral), SKIN and SLEEP.

It is also sold as a food supplement.

## CHARCOAL Vegetable Charcoal, Activated Charcoal

Charcoal is prepared from sawdust, peat, wood and coconut shells and is used as an adsorbent in the treatment of poisoning by overdose of drugs, and in dressings as a deodorant for foul-smelling wounds and ulcers. It is used as a purifying and decolorising agent, and also in odour-control insoles and in respirators as a protective against toxic gases.

It is available as tablets and biscuits for its purifying properties and as an aid to digestion.

See Product Index for INDIGESTION.

## CHICKWEED                     Stellaria media (Carophyllaceae)

A common weed that grows everywhere.

The whole herb is used, which contains saponin glycosides, coumarins, flavonoids and vitamin C*.

Chickweed is demulcent, emollient, antipruritic, antiscorbutic, expectorant, refrigerant, anti-obese, antirheumatic and a mild laxative, and has long been used for skin conditions, rheumatism and inflamed joints.

See Product Index for SKIN. It is also sold as a food supplement.

## CHILLIES – see CAPSICUM

## CHITOSAN

This is a form of fibre obtained from the shells of some species of shellfish. It is non-digestible and hence has no calories and so is marketed as a slimmimg aid for its so-called fat-busting qualities. It primarily influences absorption of fat in the stomach and small bowel, by binding to the bile acids, which results in decreased fat absorption. It is recommended that at least 6–8 cups of water daily should be taken whilst increasing fibre intake with products such as chitosan.

Products containing chitosan should not be taken by those allergic to shellfish, nor if pregnant or breast-feeding. It is sold as a food supplement.

## CHLOROPHYLL

Chlorophyll is the green-colouring matter of plants; it acts as a catalyst, speeding up reactions, and is contained in most herbs. It is also an oxidant in body metabolism and so enhances the effect of vitamins* and minerals*. It promotes granulation tissue in wound-healing. Chlorophyll is used for halitosis (bad breath), gastritis, sore throat, and mouth and skin conditions that are slow to heal.

See Product Index for VITAMINS, MINERALS and TONICS.

It is also sold as a food supplement.

## CHOLINE

Choline is found in a number of plants, including comfrey*, dandelion* and valerian*. It is contained in lecithin* and is an essential factor in human nutrition, although it is not strictly classified as a vitamin. Choline functions as a methyl donor in metabolic processes; it is a vital component of the phospholipids found in all cell walls, and is involved in cell growth and function. It is also involved in the emulsification of fat during digestion and in metabolism of fat in the liver. Choline has been given to patients with disorders associated with cholinergic activity in the brain, such as ataxia, Alzheimer's disease and Huntington's chorea. This area of research continues. Choline is sold as a food supplement.

## CHONDROITIN

A mucopolysaccharide which is a constituent of most mammalian cartilaginous tissues, it is thought to work by attracting fluid into the cartilage, so improving its shock-absorbing capacity. Production of chondroitin by the body reduces with age, causing stiff, inflamed joints.

Chondroitin is used in combination with glucosamine* in preparations for the treatment of arthritic problems and is sold as a food supplement.

**CHROMIUM** – see MINERALS

**CINCHONA** Jesuit's Bark     *Cinchona pubescens* (Rubiaceae)

This tree is native to tropical America but is now also grown in parts of Africa and Asia.

Cinchona is named after the Countess of Chinchon (1576–1639), vicereine of Peru, who introduced the drug to Spain, after being cured of a fever by the powdered bark.

The dried bark and root contain alkaloids, which are antiseptic and febrifuge, including quinine which is used in the treatment of malaria. It is also a bitter and has astringent properties. Quinine is also available on prescription for the treatment of night cramp in the legs.

See Product Index for INDIGESTION and VITAMINS, MINERALS and TONICS.

**CINNABAR**

A mineral sulphide of mercury which, when used as a pigment, is called vermilion.

Cinnabar is used in homoeopathic and anthroposophical medicine.

See Product Index for COLDS.

**CINNAMON**     *Cinnamonium zeylanicum* (Lauraceae)

An evergreen tree from Sri Lanka and southern India.

The dried inner bark of the shoots of coppiced trees contain a volatile oil, aldehydes, eugenol*, tannins, coumarin and terpenes. The leaf oil has a higher content of eugenol.

Powdered cinnamon and cinnamon oil are aromatic, carminative, stimulant and slightly astringent, also antiseptic, antimicrobial, anti-emetic and antidiarrhoeal, and are used for digestive disorders but mainly as flavouring agents.

The essential oil is used in aromatherapy.

See Product Index for COLDS and INDIGESTION.

## CITRIC ACID

Present in citrus fruit, citric acid is used in effervescing mixtures, granules and tablets. It is used to enhance the effectiveness of antioxidants, and in preparations for digestive disorders.

See Product Index for COLDS, INDIGESTION, SKIN and URINARY TRACT.

## CITRONELLA                *Cymbopogon winterianus* (Gramineae)

An aromatic perennial grass which grows in the tropics and warm, temperate regions.

The lemon-scented oil is obtained by distillation of the leaves.

Citronella oil is used as an insect repellant and as a perfume for soaps and brilliantines.

See Product Index for SKIN.

## CLIVERS Cleavers, Goosegrass        *Galium aparine* (Rubiaceae)

This common wild plant contains anthroquinones, flavonoids, iridoids and polyphenolic acids.

Clivers is alternative, antiscorbutic, anti-obese, diaphoretic, hepatic and laxative. It acts on the lymphatic system and is also diuretic, astringent, tonic and anti-inflammatory, and is used in herbal medicine to treat enlarged lymph nodes and for urinary disorders.

See Product Index for PAIN (Oral), SKIN, STRESS and URINARY TRACT.

## CLOVE                          *Eugenia carophyllus* (Myrtaceae)

This small evergreen tree is native to the Molucca Islands but is now grown elsewhere in the tropics. The dried flower-buds contain a volatile oil, which consists mainly of eugenol*. It also contains flavonoids and sterols.

Clove oil is an aromatic, stimulant, antispasmodic, anti-emetic, carminative, and is sometimes used to treat colic. It is also antibiotic and antimicrobial. Applied externally it is irritant, rubefacient and slightly analgesic. Clove oil is used for toothache, and is mixed with zinc oxide* as a temporary anodyne dental filling. It is also used as a flavouring agent and has preservative properties. Because of its antihistamine actions, clove oil can be used for insect bites and stings. It is also insecticidal and insect repellent.

The essential oil is used in aromatherapy.

See Product Index for COLDS, CONSTIPATION, DIARRHOEA, MOUTH, NAUSEA, PAIN (Topical) and SKIN.

## CLOVER Red Clover          *Trifolium pratense* (Leguminosae)

A common wild plant which grows anywhere.

The flower-heads are used, which contain flavonoids, isoflavones, resins, coumarins, minerals and vitamins.

Clover is an antibiotic immune stimulant, and is astringent, diuretic and expectorant, antispasmodic, alternative, sedative, antipruritic and anti-inflammatory, and is used for coughs and bronchitis, mouth ulcers and sore throat, skin diseases such as eczema and psoriasis, and for wounds that are slow to heal.

It should not be used in pregnancy, while breast-feeding or for children because of the isoflavones it contains, which have hormonal properties, see phytoestrogens*.

It should not be taken by those who have, or have had in the past, an oestrogen-dependent (that is, oestrogen-receptor-positive) tumour such as breast, endometrial, cervical or ovarian cancer, as evidence of safety is not yet proven.

It is sold as a food supplement.

## CLUB MOSS Lycopodium,          *Lycopodium clavatum*
## Vegetable Sulphur          (Lycopodiaceae)

This evergreen perennial grows widely in central and northern Europe, including Britain.

The plant and its spores contain alkaloids, mainly lycopodine, with clavatine, clavatoxine, nicotine and many others. Club moss also contains polyphenolic acids, flavonoids and triterpenes.

The spores are diuretic, nervine and aperient, and the fresh plant is stomachic and diuretic. Club moss is sedative and has been used for urinary disorders and in the treatment of spasmodic retention of urine, for cystitis and chronic kidney disorders, as well as in indigestion and gastritis. It is little used in herbal medicine nowadays, but is widely used in homoeopathic medicine.

See Product Index for CONSTIPATION, INDIGESTION, PAIN (Oral), SLEEP, STRESS and ADDENDA for WOMEN only.

## COAL TAR

This is obtained by the destructive distillation of bituminous coal and is a mixture of benzene, naphthalene, phenols and pitch.

Coal tar is antipruritic, soothing and antiseptic. It can cause photosensitivity and there is an increased risk of skin carcinoma with high exposure to coal tar, especially if used in conjunction with ultraviolet radiation therapy. However, it is considered that the benefits in its use for skin complaints outway the risks, and that careful surveillance and early detection result in extremely limited morbidity.

It is used to treat eczema, psoriasis and other skin disorders, in creams, ointments, pastes, lotions and shampoos.

See Product Index for HAIR & SCALP and SKIN.

## COBALAMIN – see VITAMIN B12

## COBALT – see MINERALS

## COCOA                    *Theobroma cacao* (Sterculiaceae)

This tree is cultivated in many tropical countries.

The seeds contain xanthine* derivatives and the alkaloids, caffeine*, theophylline*, and its isomer, theobromine, which has a similar, though less powerful, action to caffeine. The seeds also contain a fixed oil known as cocoa butter, or theobroma oil, as well as many flavour compounds. It is nutritive, stimulant and diuretic. Cocoa powder comprises the roasted seeds with some of the fat removed which are then finely ground. This, together with cocoa butter, is used to make chocolate and the beverage cocoa. Cocoa butter is also used to make emollient ointments and suppositories.

## COCONUT                    *Cocos nucifera* (Palmae)

The coconut palm grows in the tropics and warm, temperate regions. The oil (or butter) is expressed from the dried, solid part of the fruit.

Coconut oil forms a readily absorbable ointment base, and hence is used in emollient ointments, pessaries, suppositories, and scalp preparations.

See Product Index for HAIR & SCALP and SKIN. It is also sold as a food supplement.

## COD                       *Gadus callarias* (Gadidae)

Cod-liver oil is a source of vitamins* A and D. It also contains several unsaturated fatty acids, omega 3 triglycerides*, which are essential food factors. Cod-liver oil used to be given to infants for its vitamin D content, to prevent rickets. Pregnant women and those likely to become pregnant should consult their doctor before taking cod-liver oil because of its vitamin A content, as high levels have been associated with birth defects.

It is now taken by many for arthritis as it eases the pain. The liquid oil is much better value for money for this purpose as a dose of two 5 ml spoonsful daily is recommended. (If you don't like the taste, mix it with a little orange juice.) Cod-liver oil capsules are virtually useless to the arthritic, as they contain so little oil. Nine one-a-day capsules contain slighlty less than one 5 ml spoonful of cod-liver oil – compare the cost!

See Product Index for PAIN (Oral) and SKIN. It is also sold as a food supplement.

## CODEINE

This alkaloid is obtained from opium* or made from morphine*. Codeine was discovered and named in 1832, by the French chemist, Pierre-Jean Robiquet.

It is an analgesic, which is widely used in combination with other pain-killers – aspirin, paracetamol and ibuprofen – and as a cough suppressant, used in cough preparations.

The main problem with its use is constipation; so it is also used to treat diarrhoea.

See Product Index for COLDS and DIARRHOEA.

## CO-ENZYME Q10 Ubidecarenone

This naturally occurring substance is involved in electron transport in the mitochondria, which are part of cells. It is claimed to be a free radical scavenger, with antioxidant and membrane-stabilising properties; too many free radicals can oxidise the cell membranes and cause disease. There is a significant decrease in the amount of Q10 our bodies produce after the age of forty, so it is taken alone or in combination with vitamins* and minerals* to boost energy. It has been taken beneficially alongside standard treatment in some chemotherapy regimes, where it reduced side effects, and also in cardiovascular disorders, including mild and moderate heart failure.

It is sold as a food supplement.

## COFFEE                    *Coffea arabica* (Rubiaceae)

A variety of species of this shrub are cultivated in many tropical countries.

The kernel of the dried, ripe seeds is used.

Coffee contains caffeine*. The quantity varies with the species and growing conditions, and is reduced by roasting. It is stimulant, diuretic, anti-emetic and inhibits sleep. It is also used in homoeopathic medicine.

See Product Index for MOUTH, SLEEP and STRESS.

## COLCHICINE AND COLCHICUM – see MEADOW SAFFRON

## COLLINSONIA – see STONE ROOT

## COLOPHONY              *various species of Pinus* (Pinaceae)

This is the residue left after distilling the volatile oil of pine trees, and contains a mixture of diterpene acids, alcohols and aldehydes with sterols and phenolic acids. It is used as an ingredient of some collodions, ointments, plasters and dressings.

See Product Index for FEET and SKIN.

### COLTSFOOT Coughwort     *Tussilago farfara* (Compositae)

Both the leaves and flowers of this common wild plant are used.

They contain flavonoids, mucilage, tannin and alkaloids.

Coltsfoot is tonic, demulcent, antitussive, anticatarrhal, expectorant and immunostimulating, and is used for coughs, asthma, catarrh, bronchitis and laryngitis. Externally it is used for ulcers, sores, eczema, insect bites and inflammation and in herbal cigarettes.

It should not be used in pregnancy or while breast-feeding.

See Product Index for COLDS.

### COMFREY Knitbone     *Symphytum officinale* (Boraginaceae)

This plant likes to grow in moist places in Britain, Europe and America. Its name is derived from the Latin, meaning to heal.

The dried root and rhizome contain allantoin*, alkaloids, mucilage and some tannin.

Comfrey is anti-asthmatic, antitussive, anticatarrhal and expectorant. It is also demulcent, emollient, astringent, anti-inflammatory, stomachic, haemostatic, vulnerary and keratolytic. Its healing action is thought to be due to the allantoin it contains.

It is used internally for bronchial complaints, gastric and duodenal ulcers, colitis and rheumatism; and externally for psoriasis, eczema, sores, ulcers, arthritis, sprains and other injuries. It is also used in homoeopathic medicine.

See Product Index for FIRST AID and SKIN. It is also sold as a food supplement.

### COMMON THYME – see THYME

### CONEFLOWER – see ECHINACEA

## COPPER

A moderately hard metal of a reddish colour. It is included in many vitamin and mineral supplements, as we need it for bone formation, growth and the immune system. It is used to make bracelets, which some people find helps their rheumatism. See also MINERALS.

See Product Index for PAIN (Topical).

## CORIANDER  *Coriandrum sativa* (Umbelliferae)

The plant is native to Europe, Africa, Asia and is naturalised in the USA.

The ripe, dried fruits contain a volatile oil, which is aromatic, stimulant and carminative.

Coriander oil is used for digestive problems and in laxative mixtures to reduce griping. Applied externally it helps haemorrhoids and rheumatism. Coriander leaves have been found to accelerate the excretion of heavy metals from the body and also to assist in the eradication of viral infections.

See Product Index for COLDS, DIARRHOEA and NAUSEA.

## CORN Maize  *Zea mays* (Gramineae)

A cereal crop grown throughout the world.

The oil, extracted from the embryos of the grain, has properties similar to those of olive oil*. Because of the high concentration of unsaturated acids, it is recommended for patients with high cholesterol level and as a high-calorie nutritional supplement.

CORN SILK is the dried, silky flower threads of corn, and contains rutin and flavonoids, allantoin*, saponins and vitamins* C and K. It is demulcent, antimicrobial and diuretic, and is used for kidney and bladder disorders, cystitis and other problems of the urinary tract.

See Product Index for VITAMINS, MINERALS & TONICS and URINARY TRACT.

## COUCH GRASS Twitch          *Elymus repens* (Gramineae)

This grass grows everywhere, including Britain. As any gardener will tell you, it is very hard to get rid of once you've got it.

The dried or fresh rhizome contains carbohydrates, a volatile oil and vitamin A*.

Couch grass is widely used in herbal medicine for bladder and kidney complaints, for its soothing, demulcent and diuretic properties. It is also used for anaemia, gout and rheumatism.

See Product Index for URINARY TRACT.


## COUGHWORT – see COLTSFOOT


## CRANBERRY          *Vaccinium oxycoccus* (Ericaceae)

This low, evergreen shrub grows in acidic boggy areas in Europe, north Asia and North America. The ripe berries contain vitamin C* and anthocyanosides.

Cranberry is a bitter antiscorbutic and is also antimicrobial. It is used in herbal medicine to treat urinary tract infections and reduce their incidence. The juice can be used to treat cystitis, but a large quanitity is needed in order to be effective. However, it is also now available in a concentrated, capsule form, which are sold as a food supplement.


## CYNARA – see ARTICHOKE

## DAMIANA                    *Turnera diffusa* (Turneraceae)

It grows in southern USA, Mexico and parts of subtropical America and Africa.

The leaves and stems contain flavonoids, volatile oils, resin, tannin, and a hydroquinone called arbutin.

Damiana is aphrodisiac, nervine, tonic, stomachic and antidepressant. It is also diuretic and laxative. A stimulating tonic for the central nervous system and reproductive organs, damiana is used for nervous exhaustion, anxiety, depression, impotence, premature ejaculation and prostate complaints.

It is used in herbal and homoeopathic medicine and is also sold as a food supplement.

See Product Index for STRESS and VITAMINS, MINERALS & TONICS.

## DANDELION Taraxacum    *Taraxacum officinalis* (Compositae)

Common throughout the world, generally regarded as a troublesome weed. The name, dandelion is from the medieval Latin *dens leonis* (lion's teeth), a reference to the strongly toothed leaves of the plant.

The whole plant – leaves, flowers and roots – are used; they contain carotenoids and lactones, organic and fatty acids, flavonoids and mucilage. Dandelion is also rich in minerals* and vitamins*.

Dandelion has powerful diuretic properties with laxative and anti-rheumatic effects, stimulates the liver, improves digestion, whilst reducing swelling and inflammation. It also promotes weight loss during dieting. It is alternative, tonic, hypotensive and antipruritic.

Dandelion is used to treat liver disorders and gall bladder problems, urinary bladder problems, indigestion, lack of appetite, and chronic joint and skin complaints, such as gout and rheumatism, eczema and acne. It is an effective cleansing and detoxifying herb.

The milky sap can be applied to warts; repeat frequently to effect their removal.

The leaves and roots are used to flavour drinks, such as dandelion and burdock. The roots can be roasted and ground up to use as a caffeine-free substitute for coffee.

It is also used in homoeopathic medicine.

Those with liver complaints should consult their doctor before taking dandelion.

See Product Index for CONSTIPATION, INDIGESTION, PAIN (Oral), SLIMMING and URINARY TRACT. It is also sold as a food supplement.

## DATURA – see THORNAPPLE

## DEVIL'S CLAW    *Harpagophytum procumbens* (Pedaliaceae)

It grows in southern and eastern Asia and is named after its large claw-like fruit.

The tubers contain flavonoids and iridoid glycosides, which possess anti-inflammatory, antirheumatic and pain-killing properties, as well as having beneficial effects on the immune system.

Devil's claw is a bitter, alternative, astringent, analgesic, anti-inflammatory, antirheumatic, sedative herb, and is antispasmodic. It stimulates the digestive and lymphatic system, and is used for musculoskeletal disorders such as arthritis, rheumatism, neuralgia, lumbago, sciatica, gout and sports injuries as well as auto-immune disorders, allergies and gall bladder problems.

It should be avoided in pregnancy and while breast-feeding, and not taken by those with a gastric or duodenal ulcer or those taking anticoagulants.

It is sold as a food supplement.

## DEVIL'S DUNG – see ASAFETIDA

## DHA (DOCASAHEXAENOIC ACID) – see OMEGA-3 TRIGLYCERIDES

## DIGITALIS – see FOXGLOVE

**DIGOXIN** – see FOXGLOVE

**DILL**                          *Anethum graveolens* **(Umbelliferae)**

It is indigenous to the Mediterranean region and is cultivated widely elsewhere.

The dried, ripe fruit contain a volatile oil, flavonoids, coumarins and xanthone derivatives.

Dill is an aromatic, carminative, anti-emetic, stomachic and anti-spasmodic herb, and is used for flatulence and infant colic.

See Product Index for INDIGESTION.

**DOCK, YELLOW**              *Rumex crispus* **(Polygonaceae)**

A common European weed.

The roots are rich in minerals*, tannins, anthroquinone glycosides and oxalates.

Dock is a bitter, alternative, tonic, laxative, astringent herb, and is antiscorbutic, anti-inflammatory and antirheumatic. It stimulates the liver, the gall bladder and the lymphatic system, and is used in herbal medicine for skin problems, mouth ulcers, boils, shingles and anaemia, and also for liver disorders, jaundice and constipation.

It is used in homoeopathy for sore throats, coughs and laryngitis.

See Product Index for FIRST AID and SKIN.

**DOG ROSE** – see ROSE

**DOG'S MERCURY**      *Mercurialis perennis* **(Euphorbiaceae)**

This small bushy, leafy plant is common throughout Britain and Europe.

Dog's mercury contains saponins, amines and essential oil and is highly poisonous if eaten. However, it is used in homoeopathy to treat rheumatism and mouth infections.

See Product Index for SKIN.

**DOGWOOD** – see JAMAICA DOGWOOD

## DOLOMITE

This mineral is calcium magnesium carbonate.

It is used as a source of calcium and magnesium and is sold as a food supplement.

**DONG QUAI** – see ANGELICA, CHINESE

**DULCIMARA** – see BITTERSWEET

**EARTH NUT** – see ARACHIS

**EARTH'S SMOKE** – see FUMITORY

**ECHINACEA** Black Sampson,     *Echinacea augustifolia*
Coneflower     (Compositae)
also *E. pallida and E. purpurea*

This plant is native to northern USA and has long been used by American Indians and is now cultivated in Europe. The roots and rhizomes are used, which contain echinacosides, alkaloids, polysaccharides, flavonoids and essential oil.

The most effective herbal detoxicant for the circulatory, lymphatic and respiratory systems, it stimulates the immune system, promotes healing, and has antimicrobial actions, being antibiotic, antifungal and antiviral. It is also alternative, antihistamine and antipruritic. Echinacea is used for skin problems and infections, boils, acne, abscesses, eczema and ulcers. It stimulates the body's immune response to colds, influenza and upper respiratory tract infections and is used in preparations for the prophylaxis of bacterial and viral infections.

It is used in homoeopathic medicine and is also sold as a food supplement.

See Product Index for COLDS, FIRST AID and SKIN.

**EHA (EICOSAPENTAENOIC ACID)** – see OMEGA-3 TRIGLYCERIDES

**ELDER** Sambucus     *Sambucus nigra* (Caprifoliaceae)

This tree is common to Britain and Europe. The leaves, flowers, fruit and bark are used. They contain triterpenes, flavonoids, a fixed oil and tannins. The berries contain vitamin C* and iron. The leaves contain a toxic cyanogenic glycoside.

Elder is alternative, astringent, diaphoretic, expectorant, stimulant, vulnerary and antihistamine. The flowers soothe irritation and are anti-inflammatory and decongestant, and so are used for colds and catarrh, sinusitis and feverish illnesses, sore eyes, irritated or inflamed skin, mouth ulcers and minor injuries. The leaves are insecticidal, antiseptic and healing. The bark and berries lower fever, reduce inflammation and have diuretic and anticatarrhal effects. The leaves and bark are used for constipation and arthritic conditions, and externally for minor burns and chilblains.

Traditionally all parts have been used, but nowadays the flowers are preferred.

The flowers and berries are used to make home-made wines.

Elder is used in homoeopathic medicine, and is also sold as a food supplement.

See Product Index for COLDS, CONSTIPATION and PAIN (Oral).

## ELECAMPNE Inula, Scabwort    *Inula helenium* (Compositae)

A native of Europe and temperate Asia, naturalised in the USA, and cultivated widely.

It is named after Helen of Troy.

The flowers contain a high proportion of inulin, a slighlty sweet polysaccharide, which is of little food value but can be used by diabetics as a sweetener. Elecampne also contains a volatile oil, sterols and resin.

This herb is anti-asthmatic, antitussive, expectorant, anticatarrhal, antispasmodic, a stimulant, diaphoretic, stomachic and emollient. It is astringent and antimicrobial, and is used in cough mixtures for bronchial complaints, and also for nausea and vomiting, hiccups and flatulence, as well as being used as a flavouring in foods and alcoholic beverages.

It should not be used in pregnancy or while breast-feeding.

See Product Index for COLDS.


## ENGLISH OAK – see OAK

## EPHEDRA                    *Ephedra sinica* (Ephedraceae)

This plant comes from America and Eurasia.

The stems contain alkaloids (ephedrine and pseudoephedrine), which are brain, heart and circulatory stimulants, antispasmodic, anti-asthmatic, broncho-dilatory, antihistamine and anti-allergic. They are vasodilatory, and hypertensive – by increasing cardiac output and inducing peripheral vasoconstriction and so causing a rise in blood pressure. Ephedra is also diaphoretic. Ephedrine is used in tablets (which are prescription only) and nasal drops. Pseudoephedrine is available in tablets and medicines for coughs.

Ephedra is used for asthma, bronchitis, sinusitis and generally for chest conditions.

Ephedra, ephedrine and pseudoephedrine should not be taken by those with high blood pressure or those taking prescribed medication for it, nor with coronary thrombosis, thyroid problems, prostate problems or glaucoma and nor should it be taken with antidepressants of the monoamine-oxidase-inhibitor type (MAOI).

See Product Index for COLDS.

## EPSOM SALTS – see MAGNESIUM SULPHATE

## EQUISETUM – see HORSETAIL

## ESSENTIAL OILS

Also called volatile oils, they are soluble in alcohol and are colourless. Present in only a small number of the many flowering plants in the world, they are responsible for the taste, aroma and medicinal actions of the plant. Except for lavender* and tea tree*, essential oils should never be used neat; they must always be diluted in a carrier oil before use. Carrier oils are fixed oils such as almond*, arachis*, olive*, and sunflower*.

A fixed oil leaves a greasy mark on a piece of paper, which remains. An essential oil makes a greasy mark but this disappears as the volatile oil evaporates. Always buy good quality oils. The price varies from oil to oil; some are very expensive. It takes 60,000 roses to produce 2.5 g of oil, whereas 100 kg of lavender produces 3 kg of oil, which explains why rose oil is very expensive and lavender is much cheaper. If you find someone selling essential oils all for the same price, regardless of type, it probably means they have adulterated them with base oil and you are not getting the true essential oil. Try the paper test described above to check.

Some essential oils are too toxic to use:–

basil, bitter almonds, boldo, horseradish, mugwort, mustard, pennyroyal, rue, sassafras, sweet flag, tansy, thuja.

Whilst others are not to be used in pregnancy:–

bay, buchu, chamomile, cinnamon, clary sage, clove, fennel, hyssop, juniper, marjoram, myrrh, peppermint, rose, rosemary, sage, thyme.

For all other essential oils use half the normal amount during pregnancy.

## EUCALYPTUS Gum Tree    *Eucalyptus globulus* (Myrtaceae)

The blue gum tree grows in Australia and is now cultivated in southern Europe. It was named in 1788 by the French botanist, Charles Louis Lherititier, after the protective covering of the unopened flower, and from the Greek, *kaluptos*, meaning covered.

The oil is obtained by distillation of the fresh leaves, which contain volatile oil (mainly cineole), flavonoids and polyphenolic acids.

Eucalyptus oil is an aromatic stimulant, antiseptic, counterirritant, decongestant and expectorant, and is antispasmodic and fever-reducing, and also antibiotic, antiviral and anti-fungal.

It is used in inhalations and chest rubs for colds, catarrh, sinusitis, bronchitis and influenza, and externally in liniments for sprains, bruises and muscular pains, and in ointments for wounds. It is also used in throat and cough sweets and as a flavouring.

The essential oil is used in aromatherapy.

See Product Index for COLDS, EARS, FIRST AID, MOUTH, PAIN (Oral) and SKIN.

## EUGENOL

It is obtained from clove oil* and some other essential oils.

Eugenol is used in dentistry, often mixed with zinc oxide* as a temporary anodyne dental filling; it is also an ingredient of dental hygiene preparations and has been used as a flavouring.

## EUONYMUS – see WAHOO

## EUPHORBIA – see SPURGE

## EUROPEAN BIRCH – see BIRCH

## EVENING PRIMROSE – see GAMOLENIC ACID

## EYEBRIGHT    *Euphrasia officinalis* (Scrophulariaceae)

This little plant grows in meadows and grassy places in Britain and Europe. Its Latin name, *Euphrasia*, is named after Euphrosyne, one of the Graces in Greek mythology. The common name refers to its traditional use for eye complaints.

The herb contains iridoids (including aucubin), tannins, phenolic acids, volatile oil, sterols, amino acids and choline*.

Eyebright is astringent, anticatarrhal, antihistamine, anti-inflammatory and tonic, and is used in herbal medicine, principally as an eye lotion for conjunctivitis, for hay fever, and also in homoeopathy.

See Product Index for COLDS, HAY FEVER and PAIN (Oral).

It is also sold as a food supplement.

## FALSE UNICORN ROOT Helionas, *Helionas dioica*
### Blazing Star, Starwort (Liliaceae)

This plant comes from the USA.

The roots and rhizomes contain helonin, saponins and chamaelirin.

False unicorn root is a tonic and nervine. It acts on the female reproductive system, and so is used in herbal medicine for menstrual and menopausal problems, infertility and pelvic inflammatory disease, endometriosis, fibroids, threatened miscarriage and morning sickness. It is also used as a tonic for digestive problems as well as for treating genito-urinary complaints.

See Product Index for PAIN (Oral).

## FENNEL *Foeniculum vulgare* (Umbelliferae)

This plant is indigenous to the Mediterranean region but is widely cultivated elsewhere.

The leaves, stems, roots and seeds are used. They contain coumarins, volatile oil, flavonoids and sterols. The oil is obtained by distillation and contains anethole.

This is a sweet, aromatic, carminative, diuretic herb which relieves digestive problems, is antispasmodic, anti-inflammatory, antimicrobial and expectorant. It is stimulant, stomachic, anti-emetic and anti-obese.

Fennel is used for indigestion, wind and colic – as in gripe-water for babies, and the seeds are used to promote milk flow. It is also used as a mouthwash and gargle for gum disease and sore throats. Fennel is used in herbal medicine for respiratory tract disorders.

The essential oil is used in aromatherapy and perfumery, as a food flavouring, in toothpastes, soaps and in air fresheners. The oil should not be used by pregnant women.

See Product Index for COLDS and CONSTIPATION.

## FENUGREEK    *Trigonella foenum-graecum* (Leguminosae)

It grows in north Africa and India and is cultivated worldwide. The Romans used the dried plant for fodder; they called it Greek Hay – the Latin word for hay is *foenum*.

The leaves and seeds contain flavonoids, volatile oil, saponins and alkaloids. A source of vitamins* A, B1, C and minerals*.

Fenugreek is demulcent, nutritive, digestive and emollient. It is also anti-catarrhal, antitussive and expectorant. It leaves a soothing, protective coating over irritated surfaces, both internally and externally; it promotes milk flow, is anti-inflammatory, diuretic, laxative and lowers blood sugar.

Herbalists use fenugreek as an appetite-suppressant and for late-onset diabetes; it is also used for digestive and respiratory problems of an inflammatory nature, and externally for skin inflammation and cellulitis. It should not be taken by pregnant women.

See Product Index for COLDS. It is also sold as a food supplement.

## FEVERFEW    *Tanacetum parthenium* (Compositae)

This plant grows wild in Britain and Europe. The name is from the Latin, *febrifuga*, meaning 'to drive away fever'.

The leaves, collected when the plant is in flower, contain sesquiter-pene lactones (including parthenolide) and a volatile oil. The sesquiterpene lactones inhibit platelet aggregation and the secretion of the neurotransmitter, serotonin – which is one of the substances released during a migraine.

Feverfew is a bitter, stimulant, carminative and anti-infective emmen-agogue. Extracts of feverfew inhibit prostaglandin synthesis, which is why it is antimigraine, anti-inflammatory and antirheumatic. It contains pyrethrins – see pyrethrum* – and so it is also insecticidal. It relieves pain, relaxes spasms, dilates blood vessels, lowers fever (that is, it is a febrifuge), improves digestion, stimulates the uterus and is laxative.

It is used for migraine (many sufferers eat a leaf each day, although this may cause mouth ulcers), rheumatism, arthritis, digestive and menstrual complaints. It can cause contact dermatitis. It should not be given to pregnant women.

It is sold as a food supplement.

**FIBRE** – see BARLEY, BRAN, ISPAGHULA, OAT, PECTIN

**FIG**                                    *Ficus carica* (Moraceae)

The fig tree is cultivated in most Mediterranean countries, especially Greece, Turkey and Spain. The sun-dried fruit comprises about 50% sugar, plus flavonoids, vitamins* A and C, acids, enzymes and laxative substances.

Fig is a mild purgative, which is emollient and demulcent, and is used as a laxative usually with senna and carminatives for constipation.

See Product Index for CONSTIPATION.

**FLAX** – see LINSEED

**FLEA SEEDS** – see ISPAGHULA

**FLUORINE** – see MINERALS

**FOLIC ACID** – see VITAMINS

**FOXGLOVE** Digitalis                    *Digitalis purpurea*
                                          (Scrophulariaceae)

The plant grows wild in Britain and Europe, flowering in June. The flowers are said to look like fairy's or folk's glove fingers, hence foxglove.

The action of foxglove against dropsy (heart failure) was discovered in the late 18th century by Dr William Withering, who worked at Stafford and later at Birmingham General Hospital. The leaves, collected in the late afternoon, are quickly dried to preserve the glycoside content (of digitoxin, gitoxin and gitaloxin), which is used for heart conditions. Digitalis stimulates the vagus nerve and so slows the heart rate. It is only used under medical supervision. It is diuretic, sedative and tonic.

The wooly foxglove, *Digitalis lanata*, is used as a source for the manufacture of digoxin, the most commonly prescribed cardiac glycoside.

**FRANGULA** – see BUCKTHORN

**FRIAR'S BALSAM** – see BENZOIN

**FRINGE TREE** Old Man's Beard     *Chionanthus virginicus*
                                          *(Oleaceae)*

This tree grows in the southern USA. The name refers to the many snow-white flowers, which have long narrow corolla segments that look like fringes or an old man's beard.

The root bark contains the saponin glycoside, chionanthin.

Fringe tree is alternative, diuretic, laxative, stimulant, stomachic, anti-emetic and tonic, acting particularly on the liver and gall bladder.

It is used for liver and gall bladder disorders, also as a diuretic and laxative.

See Product Index for INDIGESTION.

**FULLER'S EARTH**

A native hydrated aluminium silicate (montmorillonite), with which very finely divided calcite may be associated. It was formerly used for whitening and degreasing sheep fleeces (fulling), hence its name.

It is an adsorbent, mainly used in dusting powders but also in creams. It is used in industry as a clarifying and filtering medium. It can be used for dry-cleaning in the home.

It can also be used in the treatment of paraquat poisoning.

**FUMITORY** Earth's Smoke          *Fumaria officinalis*
                                          *(Papaveraceae)*

A common plant in Britain and Europe, it flowers throughout the summer. The name refers to the diffuse grey-green foliage of the plant.

The flowering plant contains fumaric acid, flavonoids, bitters and isoquinoline alkaloids.

Fumitory is a bitter, tonic herb used in herbal medicine for its diuretic and laxative effects, and is also diaphoretic, antispasmodic, anti-inflammatory and stimulates the liver.

It is used for biliary colic and migraine with digestive disturbances. Fumitory is used both externally and internally for skin complaints such as eczema and other dry skin conditions, and is used in homoeopathic medicine.

It should not be taken internally in pregnancy and while breast-feeding.

See Product Index for COLDS, SKIN and VITAMINS, MINERALS & TONICS.

## GAMOLENIC ACID Gamma Linoleic Acid

A polyunsaturated acid, which is an essential building block for a wide variety of substances in the body, including prostaglandins. It is present in breast milk. The body produces it from linoleic acid, present in food as an essential fatty acid. It is vital to cell growth and structure. Gamolenic acid is found in borage (starflower), evening primrose, sunflower and blackcurrant seed oils. Starflower oil is the richest plant source, having over twice as much gamolenic acid as evening primrose oil.

Gamolenic acid helps lower blood pressure and prevents cholesterol build-up in the blood and is used for skin complaints, premenstrual syndrome, mastalgia, menopausal symptoms, rheumatoid arthritis, eczema, schizophrenia and multiple sclerosis.

It can precipitate symptoms of undiagnosed temporal lobe epilepsy and should be used with caution by those with a history of epilepsy or those taking epileptogenic drugs, in particular the phenothiazines, for example, chlorpromazine. Such patients should consult their doctor before taking gamolenic acid, no matter which herbal source is used.

Hypersensitivity reactions may occur. It is sold as a food supplement.

## GARLIC                              *Allium sativum* (Lilliaceae)

Garlic is a member of the onion family and is cultivated worldwide. The old English name was *garleac* meaning 'spear leek', the spears being the cloves of the bulb.

The fresh or dried bulbs contain a volatile oil (which includes the sulphur-containing compounds allicin and alliin, responsible for the characteristic smell of garlic), amino acids, and ajoene as well as iodine*, selenium, sulphur, B-group vitamins* and other minerals*, including the trace element germanium. When the cloves of garlic are crushed, alliin is converted to allicin by the action of an enzyme, allinase, which is also present. Garlic is antimicrobial, antibiotic, antifungal and antiviral, and so wards off or clears infections. It is an immune stimulant, and is alternative, anticatarrhal, antitussive, expectorant and decongestant. It lowers fever by increased perspiration (diaphoresis), is a cardiac stimulant, antihistamine and anticoagulant. Garlic is diuretic, anti-obese and antioxidant. It reduces blood pressure, cholesterol and blood sugar levels. Allicin is believed to be important in garlic's protective role in coronary heart disease, as it reduces the levels of triglycerides and cholesterol. It increases the levels of high density lipoproteins (HDLs), which are thought to enhance removal of cholesterol, whilst lowering the less desirable low density lipoproteins (LDLs). Garlic is also rubefacient and insect-repellent.

Garlic is used to prevent infection and to treat colds, influenza, bronchitis, coughs and sinusitis. In Germany it is available on prescription to manage high cholesterol and hypertension. Externally it is used for skin problems, such as acne and for fungal infections.

Recent research has found that allicin is effective against the so-called 'superbug' methicillin-resistant staphylococcus aureus (MRSA), even in very dilute solution. It has been tried on hospital patients infected with MRSA, as a cream, with no adverse effects.

It should not be taken by those with clotting disorders, those taking anticoagulants or those awaiting surgery.

See Product Index for COLDS. It is also sold as a food supplement.

## GELATIN

A purified protein obtained by processing animal cartilaginous tissue, such as skin, tendons, ligaments and bones in boiling water.

It is used as a nutrient and is taken daily by those with brittle nails. It is used as an ingredient in the preparation of pastes, pastilles, pessaries and suppositories. It is the main ingredient of capsules shells, although a new vegetable-based capsule is now available.

## GELSEMIUM  *Gelsemium sempervirens* (Loganiaceae)

This plant grows in the southern USA.

The root or rhizome contains alkaloids, iridoids, coumarins and tannins.

Gelsemium is sedative, antispasmodic, analgesic, diaphoretic and reduces fevers. It is used mainly for neuralgic conditions, such as trigeminal neuralgia and migraine.

It is used in homoeopathic medicine.

See Product Index for COLDS, HAY FEVER, PAIN (Oral), and STRESS.

## GENTIAN                    *Gentiana lutea* (Gentianaceae)

This yellow-flowered plant grows in the mountainous parts of Europe. Gentius, King of Ancient Illyria is said to have discovered the medicinal properties of the roots.

The dried rhizomes and roots contain xanthones, iridoids, alkaloids, phenolic acids, pectin* and gum, but no tannin.

Gentian is a very bitter, carminative, hepatic, tonic herb, which helps the digestive system, stimulating gastric secretions and the appetite, and protecting against indigestion. It also is antimicrobial, anti-inflammatory, analgesic and reduces fever, as well as being used to treat nausea, vomiting and travel sickness.

Gentian should not be taken in pregnancy or by those with gastric ulcers.

It is used in homoeopathic medicine.

See Product Index for INDIGESTION, SLEEP and STRESS.


## GERANIUM – see ROSEGERANIUM


## GERMAN CHAMOMILE – see MATRICARIA


## GINGER Jamaican Ginger          *Zingiber officinale*
                                    (Zingiberaceae)

Native to South-East Asia but cultivated in other tropical regions throughout the world.

The dried rhizome contains phenolic compounds, gingerols, mucilage and volatile oil.

Ginger root is diaphoretic, anti-inflammatory, carminative, antispasmodic, anticatarrhal, expectorant, anticholesterol and anti-emetic. It is a circulatory stimulant that improves digestion and liver function by improving the production and secretion of bile, aiding fat breakdown and lowering cholesterol levels, so speeding up the digestive process and relieving intestinal spasm, flatulence and pain.

A natural remedy for nausea, vomiting, travel sickness and morning sickness, also for indigestion, colic, coughs, colds, influenza and peripheral circulatory disorders. It is also used as a flavouring and is an important culinary spice, both fresh and dried.

It is used in homoeopathic medicine. The essential oil is used in aromatherapy.

Ginger should not be taken by those with inflammatory skin conditions, gastric ulcers or high fever.

See Product Index for INDIGESTION and NAUSEA. It is also sold as a food supplement.

### GINKGO Maidenhair Tree      *Ginkgo biloba* (Ginkgoaceae)

A fossil tree, the oldest living tree species, ginkgo is indigenous to China and Japan, now cultivated elsewhere. The Chinese name is *yinxing*, meaning 'silver apricot'.

The seeds and leaves contain terpenes, tannins, lignans, flavonoids and ginkgolides A, B and C, of which B is the most potent. It acts as a platelet-activating-factor blocker, and inhibits allergic response.

Ginkgo is a circulatory stimulant and energy enhancer, and dilates the bronchi and blood vessels, controls allergic responses and has antidepressant, antibacterial and antifungal properties. It is used for circulatory problems to the extremities (hands and feet), such as Raynaud's disease and varicose veins, also for asthma, coughs and urinary incontinence. It may help the blood flow to the brain as in cerebral insufficiency of old age and the early stages of Alzheimer's disease. Ginkgolides have been investigated for the management of asthma and for various inflammatory and immune disorders, as well as tinnitus and dizziness.

It may take up to 12 weeks of regular use before maximum benefit is realised.

Due the its platelet-activating-factor blocking action, Ginkgo should not be taken by those who are taking anticoagulants, or aspirin, without their doctor's approval, nor by those taking medication for high blood pressure. It should not be taken by patients taking thiazide diuretics, for example, bendrofluazide, or those who use migraine remedies containing ergotamine.

It is used in homoeopathic medicine and is sold as a food supplement.

## GINSENG, CHINESE *Panax ginseng* (Araliaceae)

Native to China and now cultivated also in Korea, Japan and Russia. The name is from the Chinese, meaning 'herb like a man' as the herb has a forked root, suggesting a human body, which resembles the Chinese ideogram for human being, or man. The Latin name, *panax*, is derived from the Greek word, *panacea*, meaning 'all-healing'.

## GINSENG, SIBERIAN *Eleutherococcus senticosus* (Araliaceae)

The active constituents are similar to those of panax but stronger.

The root contains gum, resin, starch, saponin glycosides and volatile oil.

Ginseng acts as an alternative tonic, and both relaxes and stimulates the nervous system, encourages secretion of hormones, lowers cholesterol and blood sugars, improves stamina, and increases resistance to disease. It is anti-inflammatory, aphrodisiac, stimulant, antioxidant and anticoagulant.

Ginseng is used to promote physical and intellectual efficiency and raises the mood, inducing a feeling of wellbeing, as a general tonic, and for fatigue and post-viral fatigue syndrome.

It should be avoided in pregnancy and whilst breast-feeding, and should not be taken by those taking digoxin* as it raises the serum digoxin level. Ginseng should not be given to children and should not be taken for more than three months without a break.

It should not be taken by those who have been prescribed monoamine oxidase inhibitors (MAOIs) such as phenelzine.

See Product Index for VITAMINS, MINERALS & TONICS. It is also sold as a food supplement.

## GLAUBER'S SALT – see SODIUM SULPHATE

## GLOBE ARTICHOKE – see ARTICHOKE

## GLUCOSAMINE

It is found naturally in the body, especially in cartilage, tendons and ligaments. It is made by the body and plays an important role in the maintenance of joint cartilage. But this ability declines with age and predisposes the body to arthritis

Glucosamine has been used in the treatment of rheumatic disorders for over 20 years, as an alternative to the non-steroidal, anti-inflammatory drugs prescribed by doctors. Only minor side effects, such as nausea and gastrointestinal problems occur, and they can be overcome by taking glucosamine with food.

It is sold as a food supplement often in combination with chondroitin*.

## GLUTEN

A mixture of two proteins, gliadin and glutenin, present in wheat flour and to a lesser extent in barley*, oats* and rye. Patients with coeliac disease are sensitive to the gliadin fraction of gluten contained in the normal diet and need to eat gluten-free foods, which are available from a number of manufacturers, either to buy or on prescription. A gluten-free diet may also help those with the skin condition dermatitis herpetiformis.

## GLYCERIN Glycerol

A trihydric alcohol made from fats or oils or by fermentation, which is demulcent and slightly laxative, employed as a sweetening agent in mixtures, linctuses and pastilles. Externally it is used for its water-retaining and emollient properties in dermatological preparations. It is used in the manufacture of kaolin poultice and magnesium sulphate paste, and in eardrops, where it softens wax.

See Product Index for COLDS, EARS and SKIN.

## GLYCEROL – see GLYCERIN

## GOLDENSEAL Yellow root

*Hydrastis canadensis*
(Ranunculaceae)

This plant is native to North America where it has long been used by American Indians for its soothing properties and also as a yellow dye for clothing and weapons.

The dried rhizome and roots contain the isoquinoline alkaloids hydrastine, berberine and canadine, as well as a small amount of volatile oil and resin.

This herb is alternative, antiseptic, antimicrobial, antibiotic, antiviral, vulnerary and haemostatic. An immune stimulant which is anti-catarrhal, antioxidant, antihistamine and reduces inflammation; a tonic which increases bile flow and uterine contractions and is mildly laxative. It also improves the digestion and is decongestant.

Golden seal is used internally for digestive disorders, catarrh, sinusitis, and excessive and painful periods and externally for ear inflammation, conjunctivitis, gum disease and vaginal infections.

It is used in homoeopathic medicine.

It should not be used in pregnancy, whilst breast-feeding, or by those with high blood pressure.

See Product Index for INDIGESTION and PAIN (Oral). It is also sold as a food supplement.

## GOOSEGRASS – see CLIVERS

## GRAPHITE

A mineral, commonly called blacklead or plumbago, although it is composed of carbon. It is used in homoeopathic medicine, where it is called graphites.

See Product Index for CONSTIPATION, HAEMORRHOIDS and SKIN.

### GRAVEL ROOT    *Eupatorium purpureum* (Compositae)

The plant grows in the USA. Its Latin name is derived from Eupator, a 1st century bc king of Persia, famed for his herbal skills.

The rhizome and root contain flavonoids, resin and volatile oil.

A soothing, astringent, diuretic herb which is antirheumatic and anti-gout and acts especially on the genito-urinary tract, including stones and gravel of the kidney and bladder, hence its common name.

See Product Index for PAIN (Oral).

### GREEN-LIPPED MUSSEL    *Perna canaliculata* (Mytilidae)

This mussel is found in the waters of the Southern Ocean around New Zealand.

An extract from this mussel contains amino acids, fats, carbohydrates and minerals and is promoted for the treatment of rheumatic disorders. It is sold as a food supplement.

### GROUND IVY – see IVY

### GROUND NUT – see ARACHIS

### GUAIACUM – see LIGNUM VITAE

### GUARANA Brazilian Cocoa    *Paullinia cuppana* (Sapindaceae)

It grows in Brazil and Venezuela.

The seeds are roasted and ground to a fine powder, which contains theobromine, theophylline*, saponins, tannins, choline* and a caffeine*-like substance called guaranine.

Guarana is an astringent, bitter herb, a narcotic, nervine febrifuge, with a strong stimulant effect – an aphrodisiac, nerve relaxant and anti-stress agent, and acts as a tonic.

It has a mild stimulant effect on the central nervous system and is taken to relieve tiredness, aid concentration and lift the spirits, but may cause sleeplessness, anxiety, tremor, palpitations and withdrawal headaches.

It should not be taken by those with cardiovascular disease or high blood pressure.

It is sold as a food supplement.

**GUM ARABIC** – see ACACIA

**GUM BENZOIN** – see BENZOIN

**GUTTA PERCHA**    *Palaquium gutta* (Sapotaceae)

This tree grows in Malaysia. The coagulated, dried, purified latex collected from the tree is known as gutta percha, and is used in a variety of dressings and in dentistry as a temporary filling material and for taking dental impressions.

**GYPSUM** – see CALCIUM SULPHATE

## HALIBUT    *Hippoglossus hippoglossus* (Pleuronectidae)

A fixed oil is extracted from the fresh or suitably preserved livers of this fatty fish.

Halibut was originally 'holy butt', meaning a flat fish eaten only on holy days.

The oil is high in vitamins* A and D, the proportion of A to D is higher in halibut-liver oil than in cod-liver oil*. It is usually given in capsules, as it is not very palatable. Pregnant women and those likely to become pregnant should consult their doctor before taking halibut-liver oil because of its vitamin A content.

It is sold as a food supplement.


## HAMAMELIS – see WITCH HAZEL


## HARTSTONGUE    *Scolopendrium vulgare* (Rosaceae)

This fern grows in woodlands and gardens in Europe, the USA and parts of Asia.

The herb contains tannins, mucilage and flavonoids.

Hartstongue is diuretic, laxative, and pectoral, and is also a liver and spleen astringent, mainly used, in herbal medicine for liver and spleen disorders.

See Product Index for INDIGESTION and SKIN.


## HAWTHORN    *Crataegus oxycanthoides* (Rosaceae)

An evergreen thorny shrub which grows throughout the northern hemisphere's temperate regions.

The berries, leaves and flowers are used in herbal medicine.

The flowers contain amines, the leaves, buds and flowers contain flavonoids, glycosides and phenolic acids. They also contain tannins and vitamin C*.

This herb is used as an astringent, cardiac tonic, hypotensive, anti-spasmodic, and diuretic.

Those already taking heart medication should see their doctor before taking hawthorn.

It is also used in homoeopathic medicine and is sold as a food supplement.

## HELIONAS – see FALSE UNICORN ROOT

## HEMLOCK SPRUCE  *Tsuga canadensis* (Pinaceae)

An evergreen coniferous tree found in Canada.

The dried bark contains resin, tannins and oil.

It is an astringent, diaphoretic, tonic and is antiseptic and antimicrobial. It is used orally for diverticulosis, colitis, diarrhoea and cystitis. It is also used as a mouthwash and gargle for sore throat and inflammation of the mouth and gums.

See Product Index for COLDS.

## HENBANE  *Hyoscyamus niger* (Solanaceae)

This plant grows wild in Britain and Europe.

The leaves contain alkaloids (hyoscine*, hyoscyamine, atropine*, scopolamine), as well as choline* and mucilage.

A powerful brain relaxant, sedative, a smooth muscle antispasmodic, diuretic, analgesic, hypnotic and narcotic, which is used in herbal medicine for travel sickness and added to laxatives to prevent griping; it is also used in herbal cigarettes and in homoeopathic medicine.

## HOLY THISTLE Blessed Thistle  *Cnicus benedicta* (Compositae)

This plant grows in coastal regions around the Mediterranean. It was originally cultivated in monastery gardens and was regarded as a cure-all.

The flowering tops of the plant are used; which contain sesquiterpene lactones, mucilage, lignans and oil.

Holy thistle lowers fever, is diaphoretic, antibiotic, an immune stimulant, antiseptic, haemostatic and expectorant; a bitter, carminative, stimulant tonic which is emetic and antidiarrhoeal. It acts mainly on the digestive system, but also stimulates production of breast milk, and is used for dyspepsia, loss of appetite, gastroenteritis, liver and gall bladder disorders, migraine, painful periods and sluggish circulation, and externally for wounds and ulcers.

Holy thistle is also used in the production of the liqueur Benedictine.

It should not be used in pregnancy or while breast-feeding.

See Product Index for CONSTIPATION.

## HONEY

Honey is obtained from the comb of the honey-bee, *Apis mellifera*. Honey is processed by the bee from the nectar of flowers; it contains vitamins* and minerals*.

Honey inhibits the growth of bacteria and so has long been used to aid healing of wounds and ulcers. It is used as a demulcent and sweetening agent, especially in linctuses and cough medicines and is reputed to be aphrodisiac.

See Product Index for COLDS and STRESS.

## HONEY-BEE    *Apis mellifera* (Apidae)

A preparation containing the venom of the honey-bee is used in homoeopathic preparations, where it is known as Apis mellifica, or Apis mel.

Those allergic to bee stings should always carry an emergency kit for self-injection of adrenaline, such as Epipen. Treat bee stings by very carefully removing the sting, taking care not to squeeze the attached venom sac, then bathe with sodium bicarbonate* solution.

See Product Index for COLDS, EYES, FIRST AID and PAIN (Oral).

## HOPS                          *Humulus lupulus* (Cannabaceae)

Hops are grown throughout Europe, parts of Asia and in North America.

The dried flowers contain oestrogens, flavonoids, tannins, resin and volatile oil.

The hop is a bitter, tonic herb that is aromatic and diuretic, antispasmodic, stomachic, antibilious and analgesic, and has antibacterial and hormonal effects. It is also sedative, tranquillising and hypnotic, due to humulones and lupulones which are broken down in the body to produce substances that have a sedative effect on the nervous system. Hops are used for insomnia, anxiety, nervous tension and irritability, including restless leg syndrome, and nervous intestinal complaints such as irritable bowel disease. Externally they are used for skin conditions such as eczema, herpes and leg ulcers, and as a hop pillow to aid sleep.

It should not be taken in depression, during pregnancy or while breast-feeding.

It is used in homoeopathic medicine.

See Product Index for SLEEP and STRESS.

## HOREHOUND White Horehound,        *Marrubium vulgare*
## Marrubium                          (Labiatae)

It grows wild throughout Europe and is cultivated in Britain. The botanical name is from the Hebrew, *marrob*, meaning, 'bitter juice', whilst the common name is from the old English for downy plant, *har hune*. The flowering tops and leaves contain marrubiin, volatile oil, tannins, choline*, alkaloids and diterpene alcohols.

Horehound is a stimulating diaphoretic, expectorant, and is antitussive, tonic, a mild antispasmodic, sedative, antiseptic, anti-inflammatory and stimulates bile flow. It is used in herbal medicine to stimulate the appetite and improve digestion, and also for bronchitis, asthma, chesty coughs and catarrh, minor injuries and skin eruptions.

It is also used as a flavouring. It should not be used in pregnancy.

See Product Index for COLDS.

## HORSE CHESTNUT Aesculus  *Aesculus hippocastanum* (Hippocastanaceae)

The horse-chestnut tree is a native of northern Asia but is common in Britain.

The seeds (chestnuts) and bark are used, which contain aesculin, aescin and other saponins, also coumarins, flavonoids and phytosterols.

It is an astringent, tonic, narcotic anti-inflammatory, and also reduces fever.

Horse chestnut is used for rheumatism and in the prevention and treatment of various peripheral vascular disorders, for example, chilblains, bruises, varicose veins and phlebitis and haemorrhoids; also for heavy legs and swollen ankles, as aescin has been shown to reduce oedema, particularly swollen ankles in warm weather.

It should not be used internally in pregnancy or while breast-feeding. Avoid if taking warfarin.

See Product Index for COLDS, HAEMORRHOIDS, MOUTH and PAIN (Oral).

It is also sold as a food supplement.

## HORSERADISH  *Cochlearia armoracia* (Cruciferae)

This plant comes from eastern Europe but is cultivated in Britain and the USA.

The leaves and roots contain asparagine, sinigrin and other glucosinolates, resin plus vitamins* of the B and C groups, and also coumarins, phenols and essential oil.

An alternative to cayenne pepper*, horseradish is an immune stimulant and is carminative, stimulant, aperient and diuretic. It is a counterirritant, diaphoretic and antibiotic, and is used for general debility, respiratory and urinary infections and fevers, for arthritis, gout, sciatica, chilblains and other circulatory problems.

It should not be given to patients with stomach ulcers or thyroid problems.

See Product Index for PAIN (Oral) and URINARY TRACT.

It is also sold as a food supplement.

## HORSETAIL Equisetum     *Equisetum arvense* (Equisetaceae)

A plant which grows on wet ground and waste places throughout Britain.

The dried stems are rich in silica, as silicic acid, and contain other minerals and alkaloids, flavonoids and sterols. An astringent, vulnerary, healing herb which acts mainly on the genito-urinary system; a soothing diuretic, which is haemostatic and stimulates the white blood cells. Horsetail is used for cystitis, urethritis, prostatitis, respiratory disorders, chronic bladder infections and incontinence. The silica in horsetail preserves the elasticity of connective tissue and controls the absorption of calcium; and is a vital ingredient of hair, teeth, nails and bones. It is used in homoeopathic medicine.

See Product Index for URINARY TRACT.

It is also sold as a food supplement.

## HYDRANGEA     *Hydrangea arborescens* (Hydrangeaceae)

This species comes from the USA where it was used by the native American Indians. The name, hydrangea, refers to the plant's cup-shaped seed capsule, which comes from the Greek for 'water vessel'.

The dried root contains gum, resin, flavonoids, iron, phosphorus, volatile oil but no tannins.

Hydrangea is diuretic, antiseptic, laxative and tonic, soothes inflamed tissues and reduces formation of urinary stones and gravel, and so is used for cystitis, urethritis, prostatitis, kidney and bladder stones, also for oedema, rheumatoid arthritis and gout.

See Product Index for PAIN (Oral) and URINARY TRACT.

## HYDRASTIS – see GOLDEN SEAL

## HYOSCINE

This alkaloid is found in a number of plants, including belladonna, henbane and thornapple. Hyoscine is used in the treatment of travel sickness and other forms of nausea and vomiting, where the main side effects are drowsiness and dry mouth.

See Product Index for NAUSEA and TRAVEL SICKNESS.

## HYOSCYAMUS – see HENBANE

## HYPERICUM – see ST JOHN'S WORT

## HYSSOP                    *Hyssopus officinalis* (Labiatae)

The whole of this common garden plant is used. It takes its name from the Greek, *hyssopus*, which may be derived from the Hebrew, *ezob*, meaning 'holy herb', as it was used to purify temples and in the ritual cleansing of lepers.

Hyssop contains flavonoids, terpenoids, mucilage, resin, tannins and a volatile oil. It also contains marrubiin (see Horehound), and is an expectorant.

This herb is astringent, aromatic, anticatarrhal, decongestant, antitussive and expectorant, a diaphoretic which reduces fever and inflammation, is antispasmodic, carminative and hepatic, acting as a tonic on the bronchial, digestive, urinary and nervous systems and is used for bronchitis, colds, catarrh, and sore throats and externally for eczema and bruises.

See Product Index for COLDS.

## ICELAND MOSS

*Cetraria islandica* (Parmeliaceae)

A dried lichen, which grows in most northern countries, and contains cetrarin, lichen acids, terpenes and lichenin and has a bitter taste.

Iceland moss is demulcent, anticatarrhal, expectorant, antitussive, antibiotic and anti-emetic. It is also stomachic, tonic and healing, and has been used in herbal medicine to treat gastroenteritis and food poisoning, also bronchitis, and externally for boils and impetigo. It is added to antiseptics and to throat pastilles for dry coughs and sore throats.

See Product Index for COLDS.

## ICHTHAMMOL

Ichthammol is obtained from the destructive distillation of a bituminous schist or shale.

It is slightly bacteriostatic and has been used in the treatment of chronic skin disorders, in medicated bandages, for eardrops, suppositories and vaginal preparations.

See Product Index for SKIN.

## INOSITOL

Inositol is an isomer of glucose and has traditionally been considered to be a vitamin-B*-type substance. However, no deficiency state has ever been identified, so it is no longer regarded as a vitamin.

Sources include wholegrain cereals, fruit and plants, in which it occurs as phytic acid. Inositol also occurs in vegetables and meats in other forms. Inositol is involved in lipid metabolism and is a vital component of the phospholipids found in all cell walls, as well as being involved in cell growth and function. It is also involved in the emulsification of fat during digestion and in metabolism of fat in the liver.

It is an ingredient of many vitamin preparations and dietary supplements.

## INULA – see ELECAMPNE

# IODINE

Iodine is a non-metallic trace element which yields violet fumes if heated. Its name from the Greek, *iodes*, means 'violet-coloured', and was first coined in 1814 by the English chemist, Sir Humphrey Davy.

Iodine is essential to life; deficiency causes the thyroid gland to reduce the amount of thyroid hormones produced, leading to goitre, low metabolism, fatigue and sleepiness. Excess iodine can cause hyperthyroidism. See also MINERALS.

Iodine is found in seafood, meat, fruit and vegetables.

Good herbal sources are bladderwrack*, garlic*, kelp*, iceland moss* and irish moss*.

Iodine has a powerful bactericidal action and is used for disinfecting unbroken skin. It should be noted that so-called colourless iodine preparations do not have the disinfectant properties of iodine. Iodine stains the skin a deep reddish-brown – this can be removed by dilute alkaline solutions, such as sodium bicarbonate*.

See Product Index for FIRST AID, HAIR & SCALP, MOUTH and PAIN (Topical).

## IPECACUANHA      *Cephaelis ipecacuanha* (Rubiaceae)

It is native to tropical South America and is also cultivated in southern Asia. In Tupi-Guarani, a South American language, ipecacuanha means 'small leaves – to vomit'.

The dried roots and rhizome contain the isoquinoline alkaloids emetine and cephaeline, tannins and glycosides, and also contain starch*, choline* and resin.

Ipecacuanha is diaphoretic, stimulant, expectorant, antispasmodic and emetic (in large doses), and is used for productive coughs and bronchitis and homoeopathically (Ipeca) for nausea. It is used as a syrup for children who have swallowed poisonous substances to make them vomit, which is considered preferable to a stomach pump.

See Product Index for COLDS and NAUSEA & TRAVEL SICKNESS.

## IRIS VERSICOLOUR – see BLUE FLAG

## IRISH MOSS Carrageen, Carrageenan   *Chondrus crispus*
*(Gigartinaceae)*

An edible seaweed which is found on the Atlantic coast of Europe and North America.

It is a rich source of minerals*, iodine*, iron and bromine and is a nutrient that is antitussive, anticatarrhal, expectorant, demulcent, antibacterial and anticoagulant. It also lowers blood pressure and cholesterol, is antioxidant, stomachic and emollient.

Irish moss is used for treating bronchitis and respiratory problems generally; also for gastritis and dyspepsia, with nausea and heartburn. Externally it is used in creams and lotions for chapped skin and dermatitis.

It is widely used in the food industry as a stabiliser in dairy products and cod-liver oil, and as a suspending and gelling agent in pharmaceutical products such as toothpaste. It is included in several products as a bulk-forming laxative for constipation and in topical preparations for the symptomatic relief of anorectal disorders.

See Product Index for CONSTIPATION.

## IRON – see MINERALS

## ISPAGHULA Flea seeds, Psyllium seeds   *Plantago ovata*
*(Plantaginaceae)*

This plant is a plantain native to the Mediterreanean region.

The husk is used, as are the dried, ripe seeds, which contain mucilage, triterpenes and alkaloids.

Ispaghula husk is a gentle bulk laxative, antidiarrhoeal, demulcent and anti-inflammatory. It absorbs water in the gastrointestinal tract to form a mucilaginous mass, which increase the volume of the faeces, promoting peristalsis and thus treating constipation, irritable bowel disorder, diverticular disease and diarrhoea. It is given after anorectal surgery and for haemorrhoids, where soft stools are beneficial. Ispaghula must be taken with plenty of fluid and not just before bedtime, due to the risk of intestinal or oesophageal obstruction, particularly if swallowed dry.

It should not be taken by patients with swallowing difficulties.

See Product Index for CONSTIPATION, DIARRHOEA and INDIGESTION.

It is also sold as a food supplement.

## IVY, GROUND                    *Glechoma hederacea* (Labiatae)

This perennial herb grows throughout most of Europe.

The whole plant is used, containing flavonoids, amino acids, tannins, sterols and essential oil.

Ground ivy is aromatic, bitter and astringent, diuretic, anti-catarrhal and expectorant. It also has stimulant, laxative and anti-fungal properties, having a tonic effect on the bronchial, gastric and urinary systems, and is used for catarrh, sinusitis, bronchitis, also for gastritis and cystitis, and externally for the throat and for haemorrhoids.

See Product Index for URINARY TRACT.

## JAMAICA DOGWOOD Dogwood            *Piscidia erythrina* (Leguminosae)

This tree comes from the West Indies and South America.

The root bark contains piscidin, calcium oxalate, isoflavones, tannins and organic acids.

Jamaica dogwood is antitussive, antispasmodic, anti-inflammatory and a mild analgesic; it is also sedative, hypnotic and a nerve relaxant and is used for coughs, nervous exhaustion, tension and stress, and in the treatment of insomnia.

It should not be taken in pregnancy or by those with a weak heart.

See Product Index for PAIN (Oral), SLEEP and STRESS.

**JAMAICA GINGER** – see GINGER

**JAMAICA PEPPER** – see ALLSPICE

**JOJOBA**             *Simmondsia chinensis* (**Simmondsiaceae**)

An evergreen shrub native to south-western USA and northern Mexico.

The nut yields an oil that contains mystiric acid.

Jojoba oil is antioxidant, emollient, detergent and an anti-foaming agent and is used for dry skin and hair, psoriasis, acne and sunburn.

**JUNIPER**             *Juniperus communis* (**Cupressaceae**)

A coniferous evergreen shrub found throughout Europe.

The dried, ripe berries contain volatile oil, resin, diterpene acids, tannin and vitamin C*.

Juniper is a bitter, aromatic, carminative herb that is diuretic, anti-inflammatory and antiseptic, antibiotic and antimicrobial, an immune stimulant and is anticatarrhal, stomachic and antirheumatic, and so is used to improve digestion and for urinary problems, rheumatism and arthritis. It is also used in homoeopathic medicine, in aromatherapy and as a flavouring in gin.

It should not be used in pregnancy or by those with kidney disease.

See Product Index for COLDS, CONSTIPATION, PAIN (Oral) and URINARY TRACT.

## KAOLIN

A native hydrated aluminium silicate, freed from impurities. Kaolin takes its name from the Chinese, *gaoling*, meaning 'high hill', from a place in the Jiangxi province, where it is found.

Kaolin is adsorbent. It is used in the symptomatic treatment of gastrointestinal conditions associated with diarrhoea, often with pectin*. It can form insoluble complexes with some other drugs in the gastrointestinal tract, and so should not be taken at the same time of day as aspirin, chloroquine, digoxin*, quinindine (a cardiac antiarrhythmic), phenothiazines and tetracyclines. Externally it is used in dusting powders; it is also used for clarification purposes.

See Product Index for COLDS, DIARRHOEA and SKIN.

## KARAYA – see STERCULIA

## KAVA KAVA                    *Piper methysticum* (Piperaceae)

It comes from the South Sea Islands of Polynesia.

The rhizome and root contain an alkaloid, pipermethysticine, and pyrones (kawain, methysticin and yangonin).

It is a mild analgesic, diuretic and antispasmodic, which is a skeletal muscle relaxant and has anaesthetic properties; it has a stimulant effect on the circulatory and nervous systems, is antimicrobial, sedative and tonic.

Kava kava has been used for genito-urinary problems, rheumatism and arthritis, and is also a powerful soporific for chronic insomnia, for anxiety and stress-related disorders, including tension headaches. It should not be used in pregnancy or while breast-feeding, or by those taking benzodiazepines due to an additive effect. The stated dose should not be exceeded as it may then impair the ability to drive or operate machinery, and also should not be taken with alcohol.

Following reports of liver toxicity from Germany in 2001, where it was widely used as an alternative to benzodiazepines, the UK government requested voluntary withdrawal of kava kava-containing products, whilst investigations were made, and in January 2003 the import, sale and supply of this herb was banned to protect the public.

## KELP AND KELPWARE – see BLADDERWRACK

A preparation of various species of dried seaweed – a source of iodine\*. It must be taken with plenty of water to avoid causing obstruction of the oesophagus.

Kelp should not be taken by those with high blood pressure, kidney disorders or thyroid conditions, without first consulting the doctor, and should not be used in pregnancy.

See Product Index for PAIN (Oral) , SLIMMING and VITAMIN, MINERALS & TONICS.

## KNITBONE – see COMFREY

## KOLA                    *Cola nitida* (Sterculiaceae)

This evergreen tree is native of western Africa and is extensively grown in the tropics.

The seeds contain caffeine\* and traces of theobromine.

Kola is stimulant, diuretic and a cardiac tonic; it is astringent and a nervine antidepressant which is aphrodisiac. It is also antidiarrhoeal.

As a stimulant it is used in tonics for poor appetite, low energy and nervous exhaustion.

It is used in the preparation of cola drinks, which may contain up to 20 mg of caffeine in 100 ml of drink.

It is used in homoeopathy to treat migraine.

It should not be taken by those with hypertension or cardiovascular problems.

See Product Index for STRESS and VITAMINS, MINERALS & TONICS.

## LACTIC ACID Milk Acid

The Latin word for milk is *lactis*. Lactic acid is found in milk, especially when it has gone sour. It is produced in our bodies when the cells break down glucose without the use of oxygen, for example in muscles during vigorous exercise, which can result in a stitch or cramp.

Lactic acid is antibacterial, antifungal and antiprotozoal, expectorant and astringent.

It is used in vaginal preparations and in combination with salicylic acid* in wart paints.

It is also used as a food preservative.

See Product Index for FEET and SKIN.

## LACTOSE Milk Sugar

A disaccharide found in the whey of milk.

Some people are lactose-intolerant due to a deficiency of the intestinal enzyme, lactase. This causes abdominal pain, diarrhoea, distension and flatulence when lactose is ingested. These symptoms can also occur in people with normal levels of lactase if too much is ingested. People with coeliac disease or other inflammatory bowel disorders, such as Crohn's disease or irritable bowel syndrome, may find that, during flare-ups, they may become lactose intolerant due to the gut's inability to produce the enzyme, lactase. However, after a period of time and recovery, which may be several months, the gut will start producing the enzyme again and the lactose intolerance will disappear. Milk and milk products containing lactose should also be avoided by those with galactosaemia (glucose-galactose) malabsorption syndrome or lactase deficiency.

Lactose is widely used in the pharmaceutical manufacture of tablets and capsules as a diluent, bulking agent, filler or excipient, and is also used in powders as a bulking agent, and in dry powder inhalers as a carrier. It is usually listed under 'other ingredients' in tablets and capsules.

It is possible, however, to find lactose-free formulations of medicines for the lactose intolerant – discuss this with your pharmacist.

## LADY'S MANTLE Alchemilla

*Alchemilla vulgaris*
(Rosaceae)

A common wild flower in Britain and Europe. It takes its name from the female complaints it is used for; it was once called the alchemist's herb because of its almost magical healing properties, as shown by its Latin name.

The dried herb is taken by mouth and the root is used topically. It mainly contains tannins and is used in herbal medicine to stop bleeding and as a menstrual regulator, and also to treat gastric and duodenal ulcers. It should not be used in pregnancy.

See Product Index for PAIN (Oral).

## LANOLIN Wool Fat

Wool fat is obtained from the fleece of sheep, *Ovis aries* (Bovidae). The name is derived from the Latin, *lana* – wool, and *oleum* – oil.

Lanolin resembles the sebaceous secretion of human skin, but is not readily absorbed by itself, and so is used in creams, emulsions and ointments, with other ingredients.

It may cause skin sensitisation.

See Product Index for EYES, FIRST AID and SKIN.

## LARCH

*Larix decidua* (Pinaceae)

A common tree throughout Europe, including the British Isles.

The bark yields a resin which is bitter, stimulant, astringent and expectorant, with a turpentine-like smell.

It relieves bronchial congestion, promotes healing and is diuretic.

Larch is used in herbal medicines for bronchial and urinary tract inflammation, and also for wounds and skin problems.

It should not be used internally by those with kidney complaints.

See Product Index for EYES.

## LAUREL – see BAY

## LAVENDER
*Lavendula augustifolia* (Labiatae)

A perennial subshrub native to the Mediterranean region which grows well in Britain.

The name lavender is from the Latin for blueish, or for washing, as it was formerly used as a perfume in washing and laundering.

The flowers yield a volatile oil, also flavonoids, coumarins, tannins and triterpenes.

The oil is obtained by distillation from the fresh flowering tops and contains mainly linalol, with some cineole and a little linalyl acetate.

It is an aromatic, tonic herb, and is antispasmodic, carminative, sedative, antiseptic and antimicrobial. It also has antirheumatic, anti-emetic and antidepressant effects, and stimulates the peripheral circulation.

Lavender is used in herbal medicine for indigestion and bronchial complaints; also for depression, anxiety, nervous exhaustion, tension headaches and migraine. Externally it is used for rheumatism, muscular pains and neuralgia, and for burns, including sunburn, and insect bites and cold sores.

The oil is used mainly in perfumery, also in aromatherapy, and as an insect repellent. The dried flowers are used in potpourris and herb pillows.

It can cause phototoxicity and contact dermatitis.

See Product Index for EYES, MOUTH and PAIN (Topical).


## LECITHIN

A complex phospholipid mixture, combined with triglycerides, fatty acids and carbohydrates, which has been used as a source of choline* and inositol*.

It is a stabiliser and emulsifier obtained from soya beans*, peanuts*, corn* and egg yolks. Choline and inositol are vital components of the phospholipids found in all cell walls and are also involved in cell growth and function. Lecithin plays a part in the emulsification of fat during digestion and in metabolism of fat in the liver. The composition varies depending on the source of supply, but it occurs in all animal and plant cell walls and is rich in phospholipids which help to reduce cholesterol.

Lecithin is taken for hardening of the arteries, stroke prevention, angina, liver and gall bladder problems (gallstones are mainly cholesterol); also for skin problems, anxiety and depression.

See Product Index for HAIR & SCALP and VITAMINS, MINERALS & TONICS.

It is also sold as a food supplement.

## LEMON                              *Citrus limon* (Rutaceae)

The lemon tree is native to Asia but is widely grown in the Mediterranean and the USA. The fruit, its juice, peel and essential oil are all used.

The fruits contains flavonoids, coumarins, mucilage, vitamin C*, citric acid* (which is antibacterial), calcium oxalate and a refreshing and fragrant essential oil. It is diuretic, refrigerant and anti-inflammatory and improves the peripheral circulation.

Lemon is used for varicose veins and haemorrhoids, and for bronchial congestion and sore throats.

The essential oil is used as a flavouring in foodstuffs and confectionery, also in medicines and as a scent in soap, detergents and in perfumery.

It is also used in aromatherapy.

Photosensitivity reactions can occur.

See Product Index for COLDS, HAY FEVER and VITAMINS, MINERALS & TONICS.

## LEMON BALM Melissa          *Melissa officinalis* (Labiatae)

A perennial plant native to southern Europe, western Asia and northern Africa.

The whole plant, leaves and lemon-scented volatile oil containing citral are used.

An aromatic, carminative, sedative herb which improves digestion, is antispasmodic, antidepressant and antipyretic. It is antibacterial, antiviral and has insect repellent properties.

Lemon balm is used for nervous disorders, depression, anxiety and tension headaches, also for insect bites and as an insect repellent. Hypersensitivity reactions can occur.

See Product Index for COLDS, DIARRHOEA, NAUSEA, SLEEP and STRESS.

## LETTUCE – see WILD LETTUCE

## LEVOMENTHOL – see MENTHOL

## LIGNUM VITAE Guaiacum

*Guaiacum officinale*
(Zygophyllaceae)

A small evergreen tree from the West Indies and the warm parts of the Americas.

Lignum vitae is Latin for 'tree of life' – so called for its medicinal properties.

The heart wood contains a resin made up of terpenoids, lignans and resin acids.

Lignum vitae is analgesic, antirheumatic, anti-inflammatory, diuretic, laxative and expectorant, and is used for upper respiratory tract infections, rheumatism and arthritis, psoriasis and eczema, boils and abscesses.

It is used in herbal and homoeopathic medicine.

See Product Index for PAIN (Oral).

## LIME Linden, Tilia

*Tilia platyphyllos* (Tiliaceae)

The lime or linden tree is common throughout Europe, including Britain.

The flowers contain a volatile oil, mucilage, tannins, phenolic acids and flavonoids.

Lime flowers are astringent, diuretic, expectorant, antispasmodic and hypotensive, calm the nerves and improve the digestion. Lime is diaphoretic, refrigerant, stimulant and anticoagulant, a cardiac tonic which is a sedative nervine and so is used for colds and influenza, for nervous tension and to aid digestion.

This herb should be used with caution in pregnancy and while breast-feeding.

See Product Index for PAIN (Oral) and STRESS.

## LINDEN – see LIME

## LINSEED Flax                    *Linum usitatissimum* (Linaceae)

Linseed is a contraction of the old English for linen-seed – flax was used to make linen.

This plant, now grown in Britain as a crop, has lovely blue flowers – a blue field is a linseed crop in flower.

The whole plant is used, containing oil, mucilage and proteins. Linseed oil is obtained from the ripe seeds subsequently clarified.

It is expectorant, demulcent, emollient, laxative, carminative, antitussive and analgesic, a source of polyunsaturated fatty acids, mucins and minerals*, and is rich in linoleic acid. Linseed is about six times richer in omega-3* triglycerides than most fish.

It is used as a bulk laxative for chronic constipation and diverticulitis – a teaspoonful of the crushed (cracked) seeds should be sprinkled over breakfast cereal each morning. Its healing mucilage is good for inflammation of the gut and respiratory tract, to soothe mucous membranes, for coughs, bronchitis and sore throats.

NB: 'Boiled linseed oil', which is used for decorating purposes, has been treated with chemicals and must not be used for medicinal purposes.

See Product Index for PAIN (Topical).

It is also sold as a food supplement.

## LIQUORICE Sweet Root     *Glycyrrhiza glabra* (Leguminosae)

A perennial herb, native to southern Europe and parts of Asia, now widely cultivated.

The Latin name is based on the Greek, *glykys*, for sweet, and *rhiza*, for root.

The root contains flavonoids, triterpenes, volatile oil, coumarins, chalcones and glycyrrhizinic acid.

Liquorice is delmulcent, anticatarrhal, expectorant, anti-inflammatory and a mild laxative. It is antimicrobial and antiviral, refrigerant, stomachic, antispasmodic and emollient. It detoxifies and protects the liver and has ulcer-healing properties. The liquid extract is used in cough mixtures and as a flavouring and sweetener in other nauseous medicines.

Excess use may cause mineralocorticoid-like effects such as sodium and water retention plus hypokalaemia, hypotension, heart problems, headache and muscle weakness due to glycyrrhetinic acid, (which is a metabolite of glycyrrhizinic acid), inhibiting the enzyme cortisol oxidase, which results in an increased concentration of cortisol in the body. De-glycyrrhizinised liquorice reduces this action and so is not usually associated with these effects.

It should not be taken in pregnancy, hypertension, kidney disease or by those taking digoxin.

See Product Index for COLDS and SKIN. It is also sold as a food supplement.

## LOBELIA Indian Tobacco     *Lobelia inflata* (Lobeliaceae)

A shrub or small tree which grows in eastern USA, named after Matthias de Lobel (1538–1616), a Flemish botanist to King James I.

The dried herb, collected when the lower fruits are ripe, contains the alkaloid lobeline, plus resin, gum, wax, lignin and fixed oil.

Lobelia is a mild sedative and relaxant, and is antibiotic, decongestant, antitussive, emetic and antispasmodic. A diaphoretic febrifuge with stimulant and antihistamine actions. It is anti-asthmatic – lobeline acts as a bronchodilator so it is used for asthma, bronchitis, sinusitis, croup, whooping cough and pleurisy, but large doses cause nausea, vomiting and drowsiness. Externally it is used for rheumatism, boils and ulcers.

It should not be taken in pregnancy or by those with heart complaints.

See Product Index for COLDS. It is also sold as a food supplement.

## LOOSESTRIFE Yellow Willowherb *Lysimachia vulgaris* (Primulaceae)

This plant grows in wet places and on river banks in Britain and Europe and is named after Lysimachus, King of Thrace, who discovered the plant's medicinal properties over 2,000 years ago.

The whole plant is used, which contains saponins, rutin and tannins. Loosestrife is astringent and expectorant and is used in herbal medicine for nosebleeds, wounds and excessive menstrual flow.

See Product Index for SKIN.

## LOVAGE *Levisticum officinalis* (Umbelliferae)

This perennial herb is native to the Mediterranean region, and is now cultivated in Britain and the USA.

The root and rhizome contain a volatile oil plus coumarins and butyric acid.

Lovage is aromatic, carminative, stimulant and diuretic, and is also antimicrobial, diaphoretic, expectorant, anticatarrhal, antispasmodic and sedative, and is used in herbal medicine for indigestion, colic, wind and poor appetite; it is also for sore throats and mouth ulcers.

The oil is used as a food flavouring and in alcoholic drinks.

See Product Index for STRESS.

## LUCERNE – see ALFALFA

**LUNGWORT** Pulmonaria          *Pulmonaria officinalis*
                                          (Boraginaceae)

This plant grows in shady places throughout Europe, including Britain. Its name derives from its action on the lungs.

The flowering plant is used, which contains allantoin*, flavonoids, palmitic acid, linoleic acid, tannins, saponin and ergosterol.

Lungwort is demulcent, emollient, expectorant, astringent and antibiotic and is used for coughs, bronchitis and catarrh; also for haemorrhoids and diarrhoea. It has also been used for wounds and as an eyewash.

See Product Index for COLDS.


**LUPULUS** – see HOPS


**LYCOPENE** – see OLIVE


**LYCOPODIUM** – see CLUB MOSS

## MACE                    *Myristica fragrans* (Myristicaceae)

An evergreen tree native to the rainforest in the Molucca Islands.

Mace is the outer shell of nutmeg seeds, and contains myristicin in a volatile oil, which closely resembles nutmeg* oil.

Mace is stimulant and carminative and is used in powder form for flatulent dyspepsia.

It is also used in preparations for musculo-skeletal and respiratory tract disorders.

As with nutmeg*, large doses may cause hallucinations and epileptiform convulsions.


## MAGNESIUM – see MINERALS


## MAGNESIUM CARBONATE

Magnesium carbonate occurs naturally as a mineral called magnesite.

Magnesium carbonate is a weak antacid and a weak laxative, which is used in indigestion preparations, frequently in combination with aluminium containing antacids, to reduce the constipating effect of the latter.

See Product Index for INDIGESTION.


## MAGNESIUM HYDROXIDE

Magnesium hydroxide occurs naturally as a mineral called brucite.

Magnesium hydroxide is an antacid and a weak laxative which, like magnesium carbonate, is used in indigestion preparations, frequently in combination with aluminium-containing antacids, to reduce the constipating effect of the latter.

It is also used as a food additive.

See Product Index for INDIGESTION.

## MAGNESIUM SULPHATE Epsom Salts

Epsom salts get their name from the fact that they were obtained from the spa at Epsom and marketed as a cure-all by the botanist and physician, Nehemiah Grew. He was granted the patent in 1698 – this was the first patent medicine.

It is a stimulant laxative.

Dried magnesium sulphate and a little phenol, mixed with glycerin, is used as Magnesium Sulphate Paste BP, as an application to boils and carbuncles; but prolonged use may damage the surrounding skin. It needs to be stirred well every time it is used as it separates on standing.

See Product Index for CONSTIPATION, INDIGESTION and MOUTH.

## MAGNESIUM TRISILICATE

Magnesium trisilicate occurs naturally as the mineral sepiolite.

It is used as an antacid and has slight laxative effects. Magnesium trisilicate reacts slowly with the gastric acid to form magnesium chloride and silicon dioxide. Thus its antacid action is slow and does not give the rapid, symptomatic relief of other antacids.

It is often combined with aluminium-containing antacids to counteract its laxative effect.

It is also used as a food additive.

See Product Index for INDIGESTION

## MAIDENHAIR TREE – see GINKGO

## MAIZE – see CORN

## MALE FERN $\qquad$ *Dryopteris filix-mas* (Polypodiaceae)

This fern is native to Europe and parts of Asia. The male fern is so-called because it was once thought to be the male counterpart to the lady fern.

The rhizome is used, which contains a mixture of substances known as filicin, triterpenes, volatile oil and resins.

Male fern is a traditional treatment for tapeworms, usually given with a laxative to help expel them. Castor oil should not be used for this purpose as this increases the absorption and toxicity, which can cause nausea, vomiting, delirium, and even cardiac and respiratory failure.

See Product Index for INDIGESTION.

## MALT EXTRACT

It is prepared from malted grain of barley* and contains 50% or more maltose, together with dextrin, dextrose and small amounts of other carbohydrates and protein.

Malt extract is used for its nutritive properties, chiefly as a vehicle in preparations of cod-liver oil* and halibut-liver oil*. It is also used as a flavour to mask bitter tastes.

See Product Index for COLDS and VITAMINS, MINERALS & TONICS.

## MANDRAKE, AMERICAN  *Podophyllum peltatum* (Berberidaceae)

A perennial plant which grows in eastern North America. In ancient times the mandrake root was believed to be like the human form and to shriek when pulled from the ground – the name is from man-dragon, *draco* is Latin for dragon.

The dried rhizome and roots contain a resin, known as podophyllin, which contains podophyllotoxin. The resin has anti-cancer and antiviral actions and is used as a paint in the topical treatment of warts. Care must be taken to avoid application to healthy tissue as it is strongly irritant. A synthetic derivative of podophyllin is etoposide which is an anti-cancer drug. This plant is used in homoeopathic medicine.

It should not be used in pregnancy, while breast-feeding or for children.

See Product Index for PAIN (Oral) and (Topical).

**MANGANESE** – see MINERALS

**MARIGOLD** Calendula     *Calendula officinalis* (Compositae)

This bushy, aromatic, hardy annual is a common garden plant in Britain.

The name is a reference to the Virgin Mary and to the colour of the flowers.

The flower petals contain high levels of vitamin A*, nitrogen and phosphorus, flavonoids, triterpenes and volatile oil.

Marigold, or calendula, is alternative, anti-inflammatory, antihistamine, antiseptic, antimicrobial, antifungal and anti-emetic; it is an immune stimulant with oestrogenic activity and a menstrual regulator. It controls bleeding and heals damaged or irritated tissues. Marigold is a diaphoretic febrifuge which is antipruritic and stomachic.

In herbal medicine it is used internally for gastric and duodenal ulcer, colitis, diverticulitis, menstrual problems and pelvic inflammatory disease. Externally it is widely used for eczema, wounds, sores, leg ulcers and abscesses, varicose veins, insect bites and stings, and dry, chapped skin and lips. Marigold is also insect repellent. It is used both internally and externally in homoeopathic medicine.

It should not be taken internally in pregnancy.

See Product Index for COLDS, FIRST AID, HAEMORRHOIDS and SKIN.

It is also sold as a food supplement.

**MARJORAM** Origano     *Origanum majorana* (Labiatae)

This herb is native to the Mediterranean but is now cultivated widely.

It contains volatile oil, flavonoids, sterols and vitamins* A and C.

Marjoram is carminative, stimulant, tonic, antispasmodic, diaphoretic, an emmenagogue, and is antimicrobial and antiviral. It is used for coughs, colds and to aid digestion, as an antiseptic and mouthwash, also to promote the menstrual flow, and for tension headaches.

The essential oil is used in aromatherapy.

See Product Index for PAIN (Oral). It is also sold as a food supplement.

# M

**MARRUBIUM** – see HOREHOUND

## MARSHMALLOW Althaea     *Althaea officinalis* (Malvaceae)

This perennial plant grows in Britain, Europe and has been naturalised in the USA.

Althaea, the Latin name, is from the Greek, *altho*, to cure.

The dried, peeled root is collected in the autumn from plants at least two years' old, and contains mucilage, flavonoids, tannins and scopoletin, a coumarin.

Marshmallow is demulcent and emollient, anticatarrhal, antitussive and expectorant; it is also vulnerary and healing, stomachic, antihistamine, antimicrobial and anti-inflammatory, and is used to soothe the stomach, cleanse and heal wounds, for dry coughs, and to soothe inflammation of the mouth and throat.

See Product Index for COLDS and SKIN. It is also sold as a food supplement.

## MATÉ Paraguay Tea     *Ilex paraguensis* (Aquifoliaceae)

This bush grows in Brazil and Argentina.

The dried leaves are a source of caffeine*, also present are theobromine, volatile oil, polyphenols and tannins. Maté is stimulant, anti-obese, diuretic and a mild analgesic.

It is less astringent than tea* and is used as a beverage in South America.

See Product Index for CONSTIPATION.

## MATRICARIA German Chamomile     *Matricaria recutita* (Compositae)

A sweetly scented annual or biennial plant native to Eurasia.

NB: Similar to Chamomile, Roman.

The flower-heads contain flavonoids, tannic acid and a volatile oil containing chamazulene, which is active against the bacterium staphylococcus aureus.

Matricaria is antimicrobial, antiseptic, anticatarrhal, anti-inflammatory, antispasmodic, bitter, stomachic and carminative; a nerve sedative which acts as an alimentary tonic and so is used for nervous, digestive upsets, travel sickness, insomnia and in babies for colic and teething.

It is also used in hair preparations as a conditioner and lightener and in cosmetics as an anti-allergen.

It may be used in pregnancy.

See Product Index for INDIGESTION, PAIN (Oral) and STRESS.


## MEADOW CLOVER – see CLOVER


## MEADOW SAFFRON Autumn Crocus
### *Colchicum autumnale* (Liliaceae)

A perennial plant found throughout Europe which produces a pale purple crocus-like flower in the autumn.

A tincture is made from the corm early in the summer, which contains colchicine (an alkaloid), tannin, gallic acid and flavonoids. Colchicine was used by the ancient Egyptians and is still used today to treat the inflammation and pain of gout. Great care is needed not to exceed recommended dose – prescription only. It can be emetic and laxative in large doses. Quercetin* can also be used to treat gout. Meadow saffron is also used in herbal and homoeopathic medicine for joint pain, nausea and diarrhoea. It should not be used in pregnancy.

See Product Index for PAIN (Oral).


## MEADOWSWEET                    *Filipendula ulmaria* (Rosaceae)

A hardy, herbaceous perennial found in moist or boggy soils throughout Europe.

The whole plant, leaves, stems and flowers are used which contain the aspirin-like salicin and salicylic acid, as well as flavonoids, phenolic glycosides and essential oil.

Meadowsweet is an aromatic, alternative, astringent, diuretic and antacid herb, which is also antimicrobial, anti-inflammatory, demulcent, anti-anaemic and anti-emetic, which soothes, heals and relieves pain. It is used for rheumatism, gout and joint pains, indigestion, flatulence and hyperacidity. It is used in homoeopathy.

See Product Index for INDIGESTION.

## MELALEUCA – see TEA TREE

## MELATONIN

This substance is produced by the pineal gland in the brain, and is involved in controlling our daily bodily rhythms, including sleep. Production of melatonin reduces as we grow older, which may explain why some people have increasing difficulty sleeping as they age. Melatonin is not available from shops in the UK but is widely sold in the USA as a sleep aid and for jet-lag and from where it can be purchased, via the internet, for personal use.

## MELISSA – see LEMON BALM

## MENTHOL Levomenthol

The name menthol was coined in 1861 by the German chemist, Friedrich Oppenheim, from *mentha*, the Latin word for mint. Menthol is obtained from the volatile oils of various species of mint – *Mentha* (Labiatae). The mint family of plants is mainly perennial and grows in temperate regions of Europe, Asia and Africa.

Menthol is antiseptic, decongestant and anaesthetic, and is used to relieve symptoms of bronchitis, sinusitis and similar conditions; it is used in inhalations and in nasal sprays, also in pastilles and ointments. It relieves itching and so is used in creams for pruritus and urticaria. It is also used as menthol cones to relieve headaches, rheumatic pains and neuralgia. It can cause contact dermatitis. As with camphor*, it should not be applied to the nostrils of infants – there have been cases of apnoea and instant collapse.

See Product Index for COLDS, FIRST AID, MOUTH, PAIN (Topical) and SKIN.

**MERYANTHES** – see BUCKBEAN

**METHYL SALICYLATE** – see WINTERGREEN

**METHYL SULPHONYL METHANE** – see SULPHUR

**MILFOIL** – see YARROW

**MILK THISTLE** Silymarin     *Silybum marianum* **(Compositae)**

This thistle grows throughout Europe, the Mediterranean region and in eastern Africa.

The ripe, liberated fruit contain silymarin – an isomeric mixture of flavolignans, also flavonoids (silibinin, silicristin and silidianin), fatty oils and sterols. Silymarin is a free radical scavenger which acts directly on the cells of the liver and has a liver-protective and stimulant effect, and is used for detoxification, gallstones, high cholesterol and as a liver tonic for 'the morning after the night before'.

Those with acute or chronic liver conditions should consult their doctor before taking milk thistle. It is sold as a food supplement.

**MINERAL OIL** – see PARAFFIN, LIQUID

**MINERALS**

Our bodies require continual supplies of a variety of minerals, which are essential to life.

Calcium     – is vital for bones and teeth, also for muscle and nerve function and blood-clotting. Vitamin D is essential for the absorption of calcium from the diet.

Chromium     – is needed for carbohydrate and fat metabolism and enhances the action of insulin.

Cobalt     – has a vital relationship with vitamin B12*, a deficiency of which can cause pernicious anaemia.

| | |
|---|---|
| **Copper*** | – is also needed for bone formation, for growth and for the immune system. |
| **Fluorine** | – is needed for healthy bones and teeth; it is also needed for muscles and blood vessels. |
| **Iodine*** | – is vital to the proper functioning of the thyroid gland |
| **Iron** | – is essential for the formation of red blood cells, otherwise we become anaemic. Vitamin C* helps the body absorb iron. |
| **Magnesium** | – is needed for energy metabolism, nerve and muscle function and healthy bones. |
| **Manganese** | – is needed in the production of some enzymes. |
| **Molybdenum** | – is needed for healthy teeth, male sexual libido and the functioning of enzymes. |
| **Phosphorus** | – is also needed for strong bones and teeth. |
| **Potassium** | – is involved in muscle function, and the maintenance of body water and electrolyte balance. |
| **Selenium** | – is an antioxidant which acts with the antioxidant vitamins* A, C and E. Men with a low sperm count should take selenium to increase it. |
| **Sodium** | – is vital for muscle and nerve function, maintenance of body water and electrolyte balance. |
| **Sulphur*** | – is needed for healthy skin, hair and nails. |
| **Zinc** | – is needed for growth and development; also for healthy skin and the immune system and in wound-healing. |

See Product Index for VITAMINS, MINERALS & TONICS.


**MINT** – see PEPPERMINT and SPEARMINT

Mint is named after Minthe, a nymph in Greek mythology.

## MISTLETOE                    *Viscum album* (Loranthaceae)

Mistletoe grows throughout Europe, as a parasite on a variety of trees.

The seeds and aerial parts contain glycoproteins, polypeptides, flavonoids, polysaccharides and lignans.

Mistletoe is hypotensive, a cardiac tonic, and is immunostimulant, anti-neoplastic, sedative and antispasmodic. It is analgesic and anti-inflammatory, a hypnotic, narcotic, nervine and is also antidepressant. It is used to treat hypertension, tachycardia, and as a nervine for certain cancers.

Mistletoe from a variety of deciduous and coniferous trees is used to treat cancer, the host tree the mistletoe was growing on depending on the type of cancer being treated. It is used as an adjunct to other cancer treatments, improving the quality of life of patients by improving their vitality, digestion, excretion, appetite and sleep. It improves mood and emotions, assists pain relief, tolerance to radiotherapy and chemotherapy and the cellular immune response.

## MOLYBDENUM – see MINERALS

## MONKSHOOD – see ACONITE

## MORPHINE

Morpheus, the Roman god of sleep, gives his name to morphine for its sleep-inducing properties.

Morphine is the principle alkaloid in opium\*, which is the dried latex from the capsules of *Papaver somniferum* – but is now more commonly obtained from the whole plant, which is harvested as poppy straw.

It is a narcotic analgesic, acting mainly on the central nervous system and smooth muscle, which is used in the relief of moderate to severe pain, especially associated with post-operative and terminal pain. It also alleviates anxiety and acts as a hypnotic where sleeplessness is due to pain.

Morphine reduces gastrointestinal motility, hence its use in preparations for diarrhoea. It is also a cough suppressant, but is not used for this due to the problems of physical and psychological dependence and tolerance which can occur with prolonged use.

Most preparations are prescription-only products; only very low doses are available in proprietary products.

See Product Index for COLDS and DIARRHOEA.

## MOTHERWORT         *Leonurus cardiaca* (Labiatae)

A strong-smelling perennial which grows throughout Europe, sometimes in Britain, named for its uses in dealing with women's complaints.

The whole plant is used; it contains alkaloids, flavonoids, iridoids and diterpenes.

Motherwort is diuretic, antispasmodic, laxative and acts as a stimulant to the circulation and uterus, as well as being a nerve tonic and sedative which lowers blood pressure; it is also antibacterial, anti-fungal, diaphoretic and anti-obese.

In herbal medicine it is used for heart complaints, and with other herbs to aid withdrawal from benzodiazepine addiction. It is also used for problems with periods, childbirth and the menopause.

It should not be taken in pregnancy or while breast-feeding.

See Product Index for PAIN (Oral) and STRESS.

## MSM – see SULPHUR

## MUSTARD White or Black      *Brassica alba, Brassica nigra* (Cruciferae)

An annual with bright yellow flowers which is grown throughout Eurasia.

The dried, ripe seeds contain the glycoside sinigrin (in black mustard) or sinalbin (in white mustard) which are hydrolysed by the enzyme myrosin, also contained in the seeds as well as a fixed oil.

A warming, stimulating herb which is diuretic, emetic, counterirritant, rubefacient and has antibiotic effects. Mustard induces inflammation, causing dilation of the blood vessels, so increasing the flow of blood to a specific area; that is, it is counterirritant.

Given by mouth, in small quantities it is used for colds and influenza, but larger doses are emetic. It is mainly used externally as poultices, plasters and as a foot-bath, for rheumatism, muscular pain, and respiratory tract infections.

Mustard is used as a condiment and flavouring.

See Product Index for PAIN (Topical).

## MYRCIA – see BAY

## MYRRH                    *Commiphora molmol* (Burseraceae)

This shrub is found in north-east Africa and Arabia, its name is from the Arabic, *murr*, meaning bitter.

An oleo-gum-resin obtained from the stems of the shrub, contains resin, gum, a volatile oil, myrrhol, and a bitter principle.

It is antimicrobial, antifungal and anti-infective; also tonic, antiseptic, anti-inflammatory, anticatarrhal, decongestant and expectorant, and is vulnerary and deodorant.

Myrrh is astringent to mucous membranes, which is why the tincture is used in mouthwashes and gargles for treatment of ulcers, also generally for inflammatory conditions of the mouth and throat. Myrrh is effective against impetigo, an infectious skin disease caused by staphylococcus aureus and, because it is also anti-fungal, it will control fungal infections such as candida. It is also used internally as a carminative.

The essential oil is used in aromatherapy.

See Product Index for COLDS, INDIGESTION and MOUTH.

## NEEM
*Azadirachta indica* (Meliaceae)

This gum-secreting tree grows in the tropics of Eurasia and North Africa; its name is from the Sanskrit, *nimba*.

The dried stem bark and root bark, seeds and leaves are used in herbal medicine. They have been found to contain at least 35 active principles, including nimbolide and nimbic acid, which are antibacterial, and azadiorachtin A, which is insecticidal.

The seeds, which contain margosa oil, are insecticidal, anthelmintic, parasiticidal, antimalarial and spermicidal. It is also anti-inflammatory and antibacterial. Recent research has investigated the insect repellent properties of neem oil and has shown that it not only reduced the number of insect bites, but also the severity of the body's reaction to them. The oil or seed extract can be used as a lotion to treat head lice as it kills not only the lice but also the unhatched eggs (nits).

## NEROLI Seville Orange, Bitter Orange
*Citrus aurantium* (Rutaceae)

This tree grows in the Mediterranean region.

Neroli oil (also called orange-flower oil) is obtained by steam distillation from the flowers of the seville orange tree. Anne-Marie de la Tremoille (1635–1722), the wife of Flavio Orsino, Prince of Nerola, popularised the use of the oil as a perfume, and so gave it its name. It is used as a flavouring agent, in perfumery and in aromatherapy. The fruit is used to make marmalade. Photosensitivity reactions to the oil can occur.

## NETTLE Stinging Nettle, Urtica
*Urtica dioica* (Urticaceae)

Nettles grow on waste ground everywhere.

The dried whole plant contains vitamins*, minerals* (iron, calcium and silica), serotonin, histamine and chlorophyll. It also contains flavonoids, organic acids and tannins.

Nettle is an astringent, alternative, stimulant, tonic, diuretic herb, and is also expectorant, antirheumatic, hypotensive, and a vasodilator, which controls bleeding, and is antiseptic.

It is used in herbal medicine for anaemia, rheumatism, arthritis, gout, urinary tract infections, allergies and skin complaints; externally it is used for haemorrhoids, scalp and hair problems, insect bites and neuralgia.

It should not be used in pregnancy or while breast-feeding, nor in diabetes or by those taking medicine for high blood pressure.

See Product Index for FIRST AID and STRESS.

**NIACIN** – see VITAMIN B3

**NICOTINAMIDE** – see VITAMIN B3

**NICOTINIC ACID** – see VITAMIN B3

**NUTMEG** *Myristica fragrans* (Myristicaceae)

This bushy evergreen tree grows in the rainforests of the Molucca Islands. In medieval times it was called *nux muscata*, meaning musk-scented nut.

The dried nuts contain a volatile oil which contains mystiricin and elimicin.

Nutmeg is a bitter, astringent herb, which is anti-inflammatory, carminative, antispasmodic, anti-diarrhoeal and anti-emetic, and a digestive and brain stimulant. It also inhibits prostaglandin synthesis and is used for vomiting and diarrhoea, indigestion and colic, and externally for rheumatism and toothache.

Large doses can cause nausea and vomiting, flushing, dry mouth and tachycardia, hallucinations and epileptiform convulsions. Myristicin and elimicin present in the oil are thought to be responsible for these effects.

The fatty oil known as 'nutmeg butter' is used in making soap, perfume and candles.

It is used in homoeopathy.

See Product Index for COLDS, DIARRHOEA, NAUSEA and PAIN (Oral).

**NUX VOMICA**     *Strychnos nux-vomica* (Loganiaceae)

An evergreen tree which grows in many places from India to northern Australia. Its name is Latin for 'nut which causes vomiting'. It is very poisonous as the dried, ripe seeds are rich in the alkaloid, strychnine, as well as brucine and other alkaloids.

It is a very bitter, tonic herb which stimulates the nervous system and improves the appetite.

It is used in minute amounts in tonic mixtures for nervous exhaustion and poor appetite.

Nux vomica and ignatia (the dried seed of *Strychnos ignatii*) are both used in homoeopathic medicine.

See Product Index for COLDS, CONSTIPATION, HAEMORRHOIDS, HAY FEVER, NAUSEA & TRAVEL SICKNESS, PAIN (Oral), SLEEP and STRESS.

## OAK
*Quercus robur* (Fagaceae)

The oak tree grows throughout Europe.

The dried bark from the smaller branches and stems are used; they contain tannins.

Oak is astringent, bitter, tonic and antiseptic, haemostatic and anti-inflammatory and is used for diarrhoea, sore throat, minor injuries and mouth ulcers and haemorrhoids.

It is used in herbal and homoeopathic medicine.

See Product Index for COLDS, PAIN (Oral) and VITAMINS, MINERALS & TONICS.

## OATS
*Avena sativa* (Gramineae)

This cereal crop is widely grown throughout temperate regions of the world.

The grain and its husk contain flavones, oil, proteins and vitamins* B and E; it is a rich source of iron, zinc and manganese. Oats contain substances which have a calming effect on the nervous system, the most active of which is gramine. Oats are antispasmodic, emollient, stimulant and nutritive.

They are used in homoeopathic medicine as a nerve restorative, a tranquilliser and are reputed to have antidepressant activity.

A colloidal fraction extracted from oats is used in the treatment of skin conditions, in the form of bath additives.

They should not be taken by those with coeliac disease, as they contain a protein (avenin) which is similar to gluten*, to which some people are sensitive.

See Product Index for SKIN, SLEEP, STRESS and VITAMINS, MINERALS & TONICS. They are also used as a food supplement.

## OLD MAN'S BEARD – see FRINGE TREE

## OLIVE                                      *Olea europaea* (Oleaceae)

The olive tree is native to the Mediterranean region.

Olive oil is expressed from the fruits; it consists of glycerides, mainly of oleic acid, with smaller amounts of palmitic, linoleic, stearic and myristic acids and contains squalene*.

Olive oil is nutritive, demulcent, emollient and mildly purgative. It is also antiseptic and antimicrobial, and an astringent nervine. It is beneficial for increasing high density lipoprotein (HDL) and lowering low density lipoprotein (LDL) in the body, which is important for those who need to lower their cholesterol level. It also has antioxidant (anti-cancer) properties.

It is used for constipation and externally to soothe inflamed surfaces and to soften the skin, in eczema and psoriasis, and to soften ear wax. It is also used in the preparation of liniments, ointments, plasters and soaps and as a lubricant for massage.

It is widely used in cooking and can be beneficial for those with high blood pressure, as it can reduce the requirements for anti-hypertensive medication. The anti-cancer properties of lycopene (the red carotinoid pigment in tomatoes) are enhanced when olive oil and tomatoes are consumed together.

See Product Index for FIRST AID. It is also used as a food supplement

## OMEGA-3 TRIGLYCERIDES

A mixture of mono-, di- and tri-glycerides of the omega-3 acids, containing mainly triglycerides obtained from the body oil of fatty fish, particularly eicosapentaenoic acid (EPA) and docasahexaenoic acid (DHA). Linseed* is a good plant source of them.

They have an anti-inflammatory, anti-platelet and hypolipidaemic action.

They are taken by those with cardiovascular disease, asthma and psoriasis, and have also been tried with some response for auto-immune diseases, such as rheumatoid arthritis, Raynaud's syndrome, Behcet's syndrome, ulcerative colitis, cystic fibrosis and some kidney disorders.

Omega-3 triglycerides are sold in capsules as a food supplement.

O

## ONION
*Allium cepa* (Liliaceae)

The onion is widely cultivated throughout the world.

The bulb contains volatile oil, sulphur-containing compounds, including alliin and allicin (also found in garlic*), flavonoids, phenolic acids, sterols, sugars and vitamins*.

Onion is antiseptic, expectorant, diuretic, carminative and anti-spasmodic, also antibiotic, hypoglycaemic, anti-asthmatic and the alliin and allicin inhibit platelet aggregation.

It is used for oedema and high blood pressure, cystitis, chilblains and insect bites.

See Product Index for COLDS, HAY FEVER and PAIN (Oral).

## OPIUM POPPY
*Papaver somniferum* (Papaveraceae)

A native of Asia, cultivated widely elsewhere. The name comes from the Greek, *opion*, meaning poppy juice.

The dried latex obtained by incision of the unripe capsules of the opium poppy, contains morphine*, codeine*, papaverine*, noscapine and other alkaloids. Raw opium, which is the dried latex, is no longer used itself, but is a starting material for a number of preparations. Laudanum is another name for opium tincture.

Opium poppy is analgesic, hypnotic and narcotic, sedative, antitussive, antispasmodic and antidiarrhoeal, also astringent, diaphoretic and expectorant, and is used in proprietary preparations for pain, coughs and diarrhoea.

It is used in homoeopathic medicine for shock, torpor, apathy, poisoning and breathing difficulties.

See Product Index for COLDS.

**ORANGE** Sweet Orange          *Citrus sinensis* **(Rutaceae)**

The tree grows in the Mediterranean region.

The oil is obtained by expression from the peel of the oranges and is aromatic, carminative, stomachic, tonic and antiscorbutic. See also Neroli (Bitter Orange).

The oil is used in aromatherapy and perfumery and as a flavouring.

Photosensitivity reactions may occur.


**ORANGE-FLOWER** – see NEROLI


**ORIGANO** – see MARJORAM

**PANAX** – see GINSENG

**PANTOTHENIC ACID** – see VITAMIN B5

## PAPAVERETUM

This is the name given to the total alkaloid extract obtained from opium, which is widely used as a pre-operative analgesic and muscle relaxant. It is a mixture of morphine, codeine, noscapine and papaverine.

## PAPAVERINE

This is one of the alkaloids produced by the opium poppy, although it is not related chemically or pharmacologically to the other alkaloids in opium and has different actions and uses.

Papaverine has a direct relaxant effect on smooth muscle and so is used as an antispasmodic in digestive disorders and for coughs. It has been used, as an injection, for the diagnosis and treatment of erectile dysfunction, but it has now been largely superseded by other agents, such as Viagra.

## PARAFFIN, LIQUID Mineral Oil

A mixture of liquid hydrocarbons obtained from petroleum.

It has been used for constipation due to its lubricant properties; however, it can result in anal seepage and so other treatments are now preferred. Externally it is used as an emollient, as in baby oil, and as an ingredient in ointment bases.

## PARAFFIN, WHITE SOFT, AND YELLOW SOFT

A purified semi-solid mixture of hydrocarbons from petroleum, also known as petroleum jelly. White soft paraffin is a bleached version of yellow soft paraffin.

It is used as an emollient and protective ointment base, including sterile wound dressings and ophthalmic preparations for dry eye.

See Product Index for COLDS, EYES, FIRST AID and SKIN.

## PARSLEY            *Petroselinum crispum* (Umbelliferae)

This aromatic biennial is found wild in south-eastern Europe and western Asia and was first cultivated in Britain in 1548.

The dried roots, seeds and leaves contain vitamins*, iron, folic acid, flavonoids, coumarins and a volatile oil.

Parsley is bitter, aromatic, carminative and diuretic, expectorant, antispasmodic, anti-inflammatory, and stimulates the digestion and uterus. It is anti-anaemic, antioxidant, antihistamine and anti-obese, antimicrobial and anticatarrhal, antirheumatic, aperient and tonic. Parsley is used for oedema, bladder disorders, menstrual complaints, indigestion, colic, rheumatism and arthritis.

It is a culinary herb which is used as a flavouring and is sold in capsules to sweeten the breath after eating garlic, onions, etc.

It should not be taken in pregnancy or by those with kidney disease.

See Product Index for PAIN (Oral) and URINARY TRACT.

## PARSLEY PIERT            *Aphanes arvensis* (Rosaceae)

An annual native to Europe, including Britain.

The dried leaves, which contain tannins, are used.

Parsley piert is a soothing diuretic which is astringent and demulcent and which is used in herbal medicine to dissolve stones of the kidney and bladder, and in combination with other herbs for the treatment of kidney and bladder complaints.

See Product Index for PAIN (Oral) and URINARY TRACT.

It is also sold as a food supplement.

## PASQUE FLOWER Pulsatilla            *Anemone pulsatilla* (Ranunculaceae)

This perennial grows in temperate Eurasia and northern Africa. It flowers around Easter time, hence paschal or pasque flower.

The whole dried plant contains tannins, saponins and anemone camphor. The fresh plant should not be used.

Pasque flower, or pulsatilla is a female nerve relaxant, mild sedative, mild analgesic, and is antispasmodic, an emmenagogue which is also antibacterial and antiviral, alternative and diaphoretic. It is used for menstrual complaints, circulatory disorders, tension headaches, insomnia, anxiety and tearfulness, and also for coughs in asthma and bronchitis.

A different species, *Pulsatilla pratensis*, is used in homoeopathic medicine.

See Product Index for COLDS, EARS, EYES, INDIGESTION, HAEMORRHOIDS, HAY FEVER, NAUSEA & TRAVEL SICKNESS, PAIN (Oral), SKIN, SLEEP and STRESS.

## PASSIFLORA – see PASSION FLOWER

## PASSION FLOWER Passiflora

*Passiflora incarnata*
(Passifloraceae)

A perennial climber native to the USA.

The dried leaves and flowers contain alkaloids, flavonoids, rutin and saponarin.

A bitter, sedative herb that is narcotic and hypnotic, analgesic, antispasmodic and hypotensive, and is used for insomnia, tension headache, stress and irritable bowel syndrome.

It should not be used in pregnancy.

See Product Index for PAIN (Oral), SLEEP and STRESS.

It is also sold as a food supplement.

## PEANUT – see ARACHIS

## PECTIN

A purified carbohydrate product obtained from the dilute acid extract of the inner portion of the rind of citrus fruits or from apple pomace. It is a non-starch polysaccharide constituent of dietary fibre. As a soluble type of fibre, it primarily influences absorption of fat in the stomach and small bowel by binding to the bile acids, which results in decreased fat absorption. It is an adsorbent, bulk-forming substance which is used in preparations for constipation and diarrhoea, and is also used as a source of fibre and as an emulsifier and stabiliser in the food industry.

It is sold as a food supplement.

## PELLITORY               *Parietaria diffusa* (Urticaceae)

This plant likes to grow on walls in temperate regions of Europe and Africa; indeed its name comes from the Latin, *paries*, meaning wall, or partition.

The whole plant is used, which contains flavonoids, and is rich in sulphur*, potassium, calcium and other trace minerals*.

Pellitory is a stone solvent which is diuretic, demulcent, anti-inflammatory and laxative and is used for cystitis, pyelitis and urinary stones. It is also rubefacient.

It should not be taken by those with hay fever or other allergic conditions.

See Product Index for URINARY TRACT.

## PEONY               *Paeonia officinalis* (Ranunculaceae)

Paion was the physician of the gods in Greek mythology; this plant was named thus for its use in medicine.

This is a common garden plant, the root of which is used in herbal medicine as an antispasmodic and a tonic.

It is also used in homoeopathic medicine.

See Product Index for HAEMORRHOIDS.

## PEPPERMINT               *Mentha piperita* (Labiatae)

A vigorous creeping perennial growing in temperate regions of Europe, Asia and Africa.

The essential, or volatile, oil, distilled from the fresh, flowering tops, contains menthol* and other related compounds, flavonoids, azulines, choline* and carotenes.

The oil is aromatic, carminative, antispasmodic, anti-emetic and decongestant, a diaphoretic febrifuge, and emmenagogue, a stimulant with antihistamine, antipruritic and rubefacient properties. It improves the digestion and has antiseptic, antimicrobial and anaesthetic effects. Its main effect is on the digestive tract, predominantly on the lower bowel.

Peppermint oil is used for morning sickness, nausea, indigestion, irritable bowel syndrome and colic as well as in inhalations for colds, influenza, sinusitis, catarrh.

It also helps itchy skin conditions and is an insect repellent. It is used in aromatherapy.

Care should be taken as peppermint oil causes irritation to mucous membranes; capsules of the oil should always be swallowed whole.

It should not be used in pregnancy, with gallstones or acute liver disease, or by those suffering from nervous excitability or anxiety neurosis. It can cause an allergic reaction in some people. It should not be given to infants in any form, unless under medical supervision.

See Product Index for COLDS, CONSTIPATION, DIARRHOEA, INDIGESTION, PAIN (Topical), SLEEP and URINARY TRACT. It is also sold as a food supplement.

## PERIWINKLE Vinca rosea

*Catharanthus roseus*
(Apocynaceae)

A small perennial, also called the Madagascar periwinkle grows as a pan-tropical weed.

This periwinkle contains the alkaloids, vinblastine and vincristine, known as vinca alkaloids, which are used in the treatment of cancer in combination with other anti-cancer drugs.

## PERU BALSAM
*Myroxylon balsamum var. pereirae*
(Leguminosae)

This tree grows in Central America.

The balsam exudes from the tree after the bark has been beaten and scorched.

It contains essential oil and resins and is stimulant, expectorant and antiseptic.

Peru balsam is used to treat catarrh and diarrhoea, and externally for wounds, ulcers, rashes, eczema and ringworm.

It can cause skin sensitisation in some people.

See Product Index for SKIN.

## PHENOL

Phenol is a weak acid found in some plants – it is also known as carbolic acid and is antibacterial and antiviral; phenol is more active when in an acid solution. It is no longer routinely used as an antiseptic, as it once was, as it causes blanching and corrosion of the skin, even in dilute solution, and other more suitable products are now available. It is not taken internally but oily phenol injection has been used to treat haemorrhoids. Injections of phenol have also been used to treat spasmodic torticollis, and liquefied phenol has been used in the past to treat ingrowing toenails.

See Product Index for MOUTH, PAIN (Topical) and SKIN.

## PHOSPHORUS – see MINERALS

## PHYTOESTROGENS

These are non-steroidal oestrogens which are widely distributed within the plant kingdom. There are several different types of phytoestrogen, including isoflavones (found in black cohosh*, red clover*, sage*, soya* and wild yam*), lignans (found in all fibre-rich food), and certain lactones (found in rye and wheat).

Some phytoestrogens, such as genistein have a structural similarity to oestradiol and so have potential to bind to oestrogen-receptor sites in the body. For this reason phytoestrogens should not be taken by those who have, or have had in the past, an oestrogen-dependent (that is oestrogen-receptor-positive) tumour such as breast, endometrial, cervical or ovarian cancer, as evidence of safety is not yet proven.

Phytoestrogens are sold as food supplements.

**PIGEON BERRY** – see POKE ROOT

**PILEWORT** Lesser Celandine          *Ranunculus ficaria*
                                      **(Ranunculaceae)**

Do not confuse with greater celandine*.

A small perennial which is common throughout Europe and western Asia.

The whole plant, including the roots, is used, which contains tannins, saponins and anemonin.

Pilewort is astringent and demulcent, particularly acting on the anus, and is used, as its name suggests, for non-bleeding haemorrhoids and itching of the anus. It can also help with the perineal damage which may occur during childbirth.

See Product Index for HAEMORRHOIDS.

**PIMENTO** – see ALLSPICE

**PINEAPPLE**          *Ananassa comosus* ( Bromeliaceae)

A perennial herbaceous plant native to tropical and subtropical America now cultivated in suitable warm areas worldwide.

The juice is anti-inflammatory; a concentrate of proteolytic enzymes from the plant contains bromelains, which are used as an adjunct in the treatment of soft tissue inflammation and oedema associated with trauma and surgery, and for rheumatism and arthritis. Pineapple is also used as an aid to digestion.

See Product Index for EYES. It is also sold as a food supplement.

**PINUS CANADENSIS** – see HEMLOCK SPRUCE

**PLASTER OF PARIS** – see CALCIUM SULPHATE

**PLEURISY ROOT** Butterfly Weed          *Asclepias tuberosa*
                                            (Asclepiadaceae)

A perennial subshrub found mainly in eastern North America.

The roots contain flavonoids, cardenolides and amino acids.

Pleurisy root is tonic, antitussive, expectorant, antispasmodic, laxative, carminative, and reduces fever, and is used for pleurisy, bronchitis, colds and influenza.

It should not be taken in pregnancy.

See Product Index for COLDS.

**PODOPHYLLIN** – see MANDRAKE, AMERICAN

**POISON IVY**               *Rhus radicans* (Anacardiaceae)

**POISON OAK**           *Rhus toxicodendron* (Anacardiaceae)

The word poison originally meant a medicinal draught or potion, especially one prepared with a harmful ingredient.

These plants come from the USA. The dried fruits contain irritant poisons, such as urushiol, which produce severe contact dermatits.

Both plants are astringent and diuretic, rubefacient and stimulant.

Poison oak is used in homoeopathic medicine.

See Product Index for PAIN (Oral) and (Topical), SKIN and SLEEP.

**POKE ROOT** Pigeon Berry          *Phytolacca americana*
                                      (Phytolaccaceae)

A perennial evergreen shrub from North America.

The leaves, root and berries contain lectins, tannin, saponins, resin and gum.

This alternative herb stimulates the immune and lymphatic systems and clears toxins. It is also analgesic, antirheumatic and anti-inflammatory, anticatarrhal and decongestant, narcotic, laxative and antipruritic, as well as being effective against bacteria, viruses, fungi and parasites.

Poke root is used in herbal medicine for auto-immune diseases, such as rheumatoid arthritis, swollen glands, as in glandular fever, for chronic catarrh and bronchitis. Externally it is used for skin complaints, haemorrhoids, and ulcers.

Poke root is used in homoeopathic medicine for tonsilitis, breast complaints, mumps, teething and halitosis.

It should not be taken in pregnancy.

See Product Index for SKIN.

## POLYPODY　　　　　*Polypodium vulgare* (Polypodiaceae)

This fern grows in Britain and Europe.

The rhizome is used; it contains saponin glycosides, polypodins, essential and fixed oils and tannin.

Polypody is tonic, expectorant, pectoral and alternative, and so is used in cough and chest disorders, as a tonic in dyspepsia and loss of appetite, and for skin disorders.

See Product Index for INDIGESTION and SKIN.

## POPLAR Balm of Gilead　　　*Populus gileadensis* (Salicaceae)

A deciduous tree which grows in Europe.

The leafbuds contain salicylates, and so poplar acts as a mild aspirin-like analgesic.

Balm of Gilead relieves pain and cough, reduces fever and inflammation, stimulates the circulation, and is expectorant and antiseptic. It has traditionally been used for coughs, colds and sore throats. The resin is one of the major sources of propolis*.

See Product Index for COLDS.

## POPLAR, WHITE — *Populus alba* (Salicaceae)

A deciduous tree found in Europe.

The bark contains salicin, populin, lignan and tannins.

White poplar is astringent, diuretic, cooling, bitter-tonic, analgesic, anti-inflammatory and antirheumatic, and is used internally for rheumatism, arthritis, gout, back pain and fevers, and externally for chilblains, haemorrhoids and infected wounds.

See Product Index for COLDS and PAIN (Oral).


## POPPY – see OPIUM POPPY


## POTASSIUM – see MINERALS


## POTASSIUM CITRATE

After absorption, it is metabolised and acts similarly to sodium bicarbonate\* in making the urine less acid, and so is used in the treatment of inflammatory conditions of the urinary tract, such as cystitis.

See Product Index for URINARY TRACT.


## PRICKLY ASH Zanthoxylum — *Zanthoxylum americanum* (Rutaceae)

A deciduous shrub or small tree which grows in Canada and the USA.

The bark and berries contain coumarins, alkaloids, tannin and oil.

Prickly ash is bitter, carminative, antispasmodic, hepatic and a stimulant to the circulation (particularly the berries). It is also a diaphoretic febrifuge, antirheumatic and analgesic, and so is used for cramp, rheumatism, arthritis and circulatory disorders such as Raynaud's disease, as well as toothache and indigestion.

See Product Index for COLDS, PAIN (Oral), STRESS and VITAMINS, MINERALS & TONICS. It is also sold as a food supplement.

## PRIMULA Primrose             *Primula vulgaris* (Primulaceae)

This pretty yellow flower grows wild in Britain, parts of Europe, Asia and North Africa.

The whole plant is used; the leaves, roots and flowers contain phenolic glycosides, flavonoids and saponins.

This herb is expectorant, anti-inflammatory, antispasmodic, astringent, emetic and promotes healing, and so is used for bronchitis and respiratory tract infections, rheumatism and gout, anxiety and insomnia.

It should not be taken in pregnancy or by those sensitive to aspirin or who are taking anticoagulants, (for example warfarin).

See Product Index for PAIN (Oral). It is also sold as a food supplement.

## PROPOLIS

A resinous exudate from the leafbuds of certain trees, especially poplar, which is collected by bees. The bees use it to make a cement to secure the structure of the hive, and seal cracks; *pro polis* is Greek, meaning 'for the city' – in this case, the beehive. Propolis protects the hive from infection.

It is antibiotic, antimicrobial, fungicidal, anti-inflammatory and promotes wellbeing, and is used for sore throat, tonsilitis and other infections.

Hypersensitivity reactions have been reported; it should not be taken by asthmatics or those with related allergies without first consulting their doctor.

It is sold as a food supplement.

## PSEUDOEPHEDRINE – see EPHEDRA

## PSYLLIUM – see ISPAGHULA

## PULMONARIA – see LUNGWORT

## PULSATILLA – see PASQUE FLOWER

## PUMILIO PINE          *Pinus mugo var. pumilio* (Pinaceae)

It is native to central and southern Europe.

Pumilio pine oil, obtained by distillation of the fresh leaves, contains esters and is aromatic, antiseptic, decongestant and expectorant, and is inhaled with steam in combination with other ingredients to relieve cough and nasal congestion. It has also been used as a rubefacient in the treatment of sprains and fibrositis.

See Product Index for COLDS.

## PUMPKIN          *Cucurbita maxima* (Cucurbitaceae)

Pumpkins are grown throughout the world. The name means large melon in Latin.

The seeds are used, which contain a fixed oil, composed mainly of linoleic acid.

Pumpkin is diuretic, demulcent and anthelmintic.

See Product Index for VITAMINS, MINERALS & TONICS.

It is also sold as a food supplement.

## PURPLE MEDICK – see ALFALFA

## PYCNEGENOL

This is a complex of about 40 flavonoids and organic acids, obtained from pine trees.

It is a natural source of antioxidants and is used to help maintain a healthy circulation and skin, and to dramatically improve skin conditions such as acne rosacea. It works alongside other natural antioxidants, such as vitamins* C and E, helping to extend their own antioxidant activity. Cell oxidation by free radicals is believed to be a major cause of ageing and degenerative diseases, which antioxidants may be able to help.

## PYRETHRUM                  *Chrysanthemum cinerariaefolium*
### Dalmation Pyrethrum                              (Compositae)

This pretty perennial herb is native to Dalmatia but now grows worldwide.

The dried flower-heads contain pyrethrins and cinerins which are insecticidal.

Synthetic pyrethroids are used in insecticidal blocks and sprays and for the treatment of head lice in lotions, creme rinse and mousse.

See Product Index for FIRST AID.


## PYRIDOXINE – see VITAMIN B6


## PYRITES

A brassy yellow mineral, iron disulphide, which is used in homoeopathy.

See Product Index for COLDS.

**Q10** – see CO-ENZYME Q10

**QUEEN BEE JELLY** – see ROYAL JELLY

## QUERCETIN

This flavonoid (bioflavonoid) and others, such as hisperidin, rutin and oxerutins, are naturally occurring antioxidants, found in many plants. In the past quercetin was called vitamin P, but as no deficiency state has been found it is no longer regarded as such.

Bioflavonoids are used to improve capillary function by stabilising cell membranes and so reducing abnormal leakage. They are given to relieve capillary impairment and venous insufficiency of the lower limbs, and for haemorrhoids. The flavonoids, which are contained in some foods, such as fruit, vegetables, tea and red wine, may have a protective effect against the development of atherosclerosis. Quercetin is also anti-inflammatory, working best when combined with vitamin C*, and can be used for allergies, such as hay fever, by stabilising the cell membranes of the nasal passages, bronchial airways and throat, so reducing the allergic inflammation that occurs. It is also a useful natural remedy for those prone to gout, as it inhibits the enzyme xanthine oxidase, which is responsible for the formation of uric acid crystals in the cells – the cause of the intense pain of gout.

Quercetin and other flavonoids are sold as food supplements.

**QUERCUS** – see OAK

## QUINCE *Cydonia oblongata* (Rosaceae)

A deciduous tree, native to the Middle East, now cultivated elsewhere for its fruit.

Also called the apple of Cydonia (now Canea) in Crete.

The seeds contain mucilage, amygdalin, fixed oil and tannins.

Quince is demulcent and has been used to treat diarrhoea and as a lotion for the eyes.

The fruit can be used to make jam.

See Product Index for HAY FEVER.


## QUININE – see CINCHONA

## RAPE Rapeseed          *Brassica napus var. oleifera* (Cruciferae)

This crop, with bright yellow flowers, is now grown commercially in Britain.

The fixed oil, expressed from the seeds, contains erucic acid; animal studies have shown that erucic acid can cause damage to muscle, especially heart muscle, and so its use in foodstuffs is restricted. Rape oil is used in liniments in place of olive oil*.

## RASPBERRY                    *Rubus idaeus* (Rosaceae)

This species is widespread in Europe, Asia and North America.

The dried leaves contain tannins, flavonoids and polypeptides.

Raspberry leaves are astringent, stimulant tonic and antispasmodic, and act to tone the uterine muscles in pregnancy, and to ease childbirth. They are also a febrifuge and galactogogue.

The leaves contain a substance, readily extracted in hot water, that relaxes the smooth muscle of the uterus and intestines, hence raspberry-leaf tea is a traditional remedy for painful menstruation and for use in the few weeks before childbirth and during labour. The tea is also used as an astringent gargle for inflammation of the mouth and throat, for minor wounds and sores. Raspberry-leaf tea can be used as an eyewash for conjunctivitis.

It should not be taken in the first three months of pregnancy and preferably only used in the last few weeks of pregnancy and during labour.

See Product Index for PAIN (Oral).

## RAUWOLFIA          *Rauwolfia serpentina* (Apocynaceae)

This evergreen shrub was found in Burma but is now grown in Europe, and is named after Leonard Rauwolf, a 16th century German physician and botanist.

The dried roots contain alkaloids, some of which act to reduce blood pressure (reserpine and rescinnamine). It has been used to treat high blood pressure, but has now largely been superseded by other agents that have fewer side effects.

**RED CLOVER** – see CLOVER

**RED ELM** – see SLIPPERY ELM

**RED PEPPER** – see CAPSICUM

**RED VINE**                    *Vitis vinefera* (Vitaceae)

Although originally from Asia, it now grows throughout the northern hemisphere.

The leaves contain grape sugar, malic acid and gum.

Red vine is astringent, diuretic, anti-inflammatory, clears toxins, controls bleeding and improves the circulation in varicose veins, piles and chilblains. It is also taken for menstrual and menopausal complaints, hypertension and high cholesterol.

See Product Index for INDIGESTION. It is sold as a food supplement.

**RETINOL** – see VITAMIN A

**RHATANY**               *Krameria triandra* (Krameriaceae)

It grows in Peru and Bolivia. The root contains tannins and so is astringent.

Rhatany root is used in herbal medicine for diarrhoea, to stop bleeding, for chilblains and wounds, and as a mouthwash.

See Product Index for MOUTH.

**RHUBARB** Turkey Rhubarb          *Rheum officinale*
                                    (Polygonaceae)

Originating in Turkey it is now widely grown. There are about 50 different species of rhubarb that grow throughout Eurasia.

The dried rhizome and bark contain anthroquinones, rutin*, tannins, fatty acids and calcium oxalate.

It is astringent, due to the tannins, and also a tonic, gastric stimulant, which acts as a laxative, as well as being antiseptic and anti-inflammatory.

Rhubarb is used for constipation, diverticular disease and gastroenteritis.

In Britain the leaf-stalks of garden rhubarb, *Rheum rhaponticum*, are used as a food, but the leaves are poisonous, as they contain oxalic acid.

See Product Index for CONSTIPATION, INDIGESTION and MOUTH.

## RIBOFLAVINE – see VITAMIN B2

## ROSE Dog Rose, Wild Rose  *Rosa canina* (Rosaceae)

A deciduous shrub which grows in northern temperate regions.

The fruits (hips) are rich in vitamin C\*, as well as A, B1 and B2 and also contain flavonoids and tannins.

Rose hips are astringent, diuretic, and mildly laxative, as well as anti-gallstone and anti-kidney-stone, and are also used for colds, influenza, gastritis and diarrhoea.

## ROSEGERANIUM Geranium  *Pelargonium graveolens* (Geranianaceae)

Originally from South Africa but now widely grown in Europe and elsewhere.

The oil is obtained by distillation of the aerial parts of the plant, and contains geraniol.

Hypersensitivity reactions have been reported.

It is used in aromatherapy and perfumery and in various preparations.

See Product Index for FIRST AID, HAIR, MOUTH and VITAMINS, MINERALS & TONICS.

## ROSEMARY Seadew  *Rosmarinus officinalis* (Labiatae)

An evergreen shrub native to the Mediterranean region, but widely cultivated elsewhere.

The leaves and terminal twigs contain flavonoids, diterpenes, volatile oil (which contains camphor\* and cineole), and rosmarinic acid.

Rosemary is an aromatic, astringent, tonic, carminative, restorative herb, which is analgesic, anti-inflammatory, antispasmodic and antibacterial, and also improves digestion and stimulates the liver and gall bladder. It is antiseptic and antimicrobial, a diaphoretic cardiac tonic and emmenagogue, and is sedative and hypotensive. Rosemary oil is parasiticidal. It is used in herbal medicine for depression, nervous exhaustion, headaches (including migraine) and indigestion associated with anxiety. Externally it is used for rheumatism and arthritis, neuralgia and muscular injuries; it is also included in inhalations and hair lotions.

It should not be taken in pregnancy.

See Product Index for HAIR, PAIN (Oral) and SKIN.

## ROYAL JELLY Queen Bee Jelly

This is a secretion from the salivary glands of the worker honey-bee. It is a special food produced to feed the developing queen bee.

Royal jelly is rich in amino acids, vitamins* and minerals* and is antibiotic, and stimulates the immune system and endocrine glands. It is used for defence against infection, for healthy skin, nails and hair, as a natural antibiotic, aphrodisiac, and to improve the ability to handle stress. Royal jelly should not be taken by asthmatics or those with related allergies without first consulting their doctor. It is sold as a food supplement.

## RUE                              *Ruta graveolens* (Rutaceae)

This plant is native to southern Europe and is cultivated in Britain.

The plant contains volatile oil, flavonoids including rutin* and quercetin*, coumarins, alkaloids and lignans.

Rue is antimicrobial, anthelmintic and parasiticidal, also rubefacient, stimulant, antispasmodic, and a uterine stimulant that promotes the menstrual flow. It is used for capillary fragility, due to its rutin and quercetin content, for oedema, and as an anti-inflammatory. It should not be used in pregnancy due to its stimulant effects on the uterus.

It is used in homoeopathy.

See Product Index for EYES, FIRST AID, PAIN (Oral) and (Topical).

## RUTIN – see QUERCETIN

**SABADILLA**          *Schoenocaulon officinale* (Liliaceae)

This liliacious plant grows in Mexico and parts of South America.

The seeds contain alkaloids, collectively referred to as veratrine and fixed oil.

Sabadilla is laxative and emetic, and is used as an insecticide.

See Product Index for HAY FEVER.


**SABAL** – see SAW PALMETTO


**SACRED BARK** – see CASCARA


**SAFFLOWER** Saffron Thistle          *Carthamus tinctorius*
                                        (Compositae)

A thistle-like plant from Asia, now cultivated elsewhere, mainly for its seeds.

The flowers, seeds and oil are used. The flowers contain flavones, which are the pigments used in dyeing the traditional robes of Tibetan monks; they also contain lignans and polysaccharides.

Safflower is laxative, diuretic and anti-inflammatory, and is used in herbal medicine for coronary heart disease, menstrual and menopausal problems, jaundice and measles. It is used externally for injuries, contusions and strains due to its anti-inflammatory action.

It should not be given to pregnant women.

The oil, which contains about 75% linoleic acid and saturated fatty acids, is used in cooking and in cholesterol-reducing diets, as with soya* oil.

It is used as a food supplement.

## SAGE
Salvia officinalis (Labiatae)

This shrubby evergreen perennial is native to the Mediterranean region and is widely cultivated elsewhere. The Latin name means 'to save', 'to cure', or 'to be in good health' – an allusion to its healing properties.

The dried, cut leaves contain a volatile oil composed of thujone, cineole, camphor* and others, as well as bitters, phytoestrogen* flavonoids and phenolic acids.

Sage is aromatic, stimulant and tonic, also carminative, antispasmodic, antiseptic, antimicrobial, antihistamine and astringent. It is used as a gargle and mouthwash for mouth and throat problems, and is also used for respiratory tract disorders, gastrointestinal disorders and menopausal hot flushes. It is used in homoeopathic medicine.

Those with diabetes or epilepsy should consult their doctor before use.

Sage should not be taken by those who have, or have had in the past, an oestrogen-dependent (that is, oestrogen-receptor-positive) tumour such as breast, endometrial, cervical or ovarian cancer, as evidence of safety is not yet proven.

See Product Index for MOUTH and STRESS. It is also sold as a food supplement.


## SALICYLIC ACID and SALICYLATES

Salicylic acid and salicylates are found in various foods: almonds, apples, cherries, cucumbers, grapes, peaches, prunes and tomatoes; also in meadowsweet*, poplar*, willow* and wintergreen*.

Salicylates are analgesic – they have an aspirin-like effect. They also have bacteriostatic and fungicidal actions and are keratolytic, and so are used for skin diseases, such as dandruff, seborrheic dermatitis, ichthyosis, psoriasis and acne, in ointments, pastes and lotions. They are used in collodions and plasters to treat corns, warts and verrucas.

See Product Index for EARS, FEET, MOUTH, HAIR & SCALP and SKIN.


**SALT** – see SODIUM CHLORIDE

**SAMBUCUS** – see ELDER

## SARSAPARILLA *Smilax officinalis* (Liliaceae)

A climbing vine native to tropical America and the West Indies.

The dried root and rhizome contain saponins, parillin, resin and oil.

Sarsaparilla is antiseptic, alternative, antiscorbutic and diaphoretic, also anti-inflammatory, antipruritic and antirheumatic, diuretic and a powerful blood tonic which stimulates the pituitary gland; it contains the male hormone testosterone and cortin, a hormone that regulates the metabolism. It has a progesterone-like action which produces heavier muscle tone and so is used by athletes to build up the body and improve performance. It is used for impotence, sexual debility and premenstrual tension as well as rheumatism, gout and skin diseases such as eczema and psoriasis.

It is used in homoeopathic medicine.

See Product Index for PAIN (Oral) and SKIN. It is also sold as a food supplement.

## SAVIN *Juniperus sabina* (Cupressaceae)

This tree grows in the mountainous regions of Switzerland, Italy and Spain.

The young shoots are used, which contain volatile oil and lignans including podophyllotoxin – see Mandrake, American*. Savin is anthelmintic, antiviral and diuretic.

See Product Index for PAIN (Topical).

## SAW PALMETTO Sabal *Serenoa serrulata* (Palmae)

A small evergreen palm found in south-eastern North America, along the coastline of Georgia and Florida.

The berries contain polysaccharides, fixed oil, essential oil and various steroidal compounds with anti-androgenic and oestrogenic properties, one of which is sitosterol.

Saw palmetto is a tonic, nutrient, anabolic and endocrine stimulant, and is antiseptic, diuretic, sedative, expectorant, antispasmodic and aphrodisiac. It is used in herbal medicine for impotence and sexual debility, in the treatment of benign prostatic hyperplasia, cystitis, and for bronchial complaints.

Sitosterol, a phytosterol contained in saw palmetto, has been used as a lipid-regulating drug in the treatment of hyperlipidaemia and for benign prostatic hyperplasia.

See Product Index for STRESS, URINARY TRACT and VITAMINS, MINERALS & TONICS. It is also sold as a food supplement.

## SCABWORT – see ELECAMPNE

## SCULLCAP Skullcap          *Scutellaria lateriflora* (Labiatae)

A spreading perennial plant which grows in North America.

The whole dried plant contains a flavonoid glycoside (scutellarin), iridoids, tannins and volatile oil.

Scullcap is bitter, tonic and sedative, analgesic, astringent and diuretic, antispasmodic, antipyretic, nervine, hypnotic and antidepressant, a brain and central nervous system vasodilator and anticonvulsant. It is used internally for irritability, insomnia, nervous and convulsive complaints, including treatment for withdrawal of benzodiazepine tranquillisers.

It should not be taken in pregnancy.

See Product Index for COLDS, PAIN (Oral), SLEEP and STRESS. It is also sold as a food supplement.

## SCURVY GRASS          *Cochlearia officinalis* (Cruciferae)

It grows wild on dry ground, particularly near the coast, throughout Europe.

It gets its name because it used to be taken for its vitamin C* content, as a cure for scurvy – that is, it is antiscorbutic. It is also a mild laxative and diuretic. It is used as a treatment for mouth ulcers and for spots and blemishes.

See Product Index for STRESS.

**SEADEW** – see ROSEMARY

**SEAWRACK** – see BLADDERWRACK

**SELENIUM** – see MINERALS

**SENEGA** – see SNAKE ROOT

**SENNA** Alexandrian                  *Cassia acutifolia*
      Tinnevelly     *Cassia augustifolia* **(Leguminosae)**

A shrubby perennial, Alexandrian senna comes from tropical Africa, Egypt and the Sudan; Tinevelly senna is native to India and is cultivated mainly in India and Pakistan.

The dried leaves and pods are used. They contain anthroquinone glucosides (sennoside glycosides). Alexandrian senna usually contains greater amounts than Tinnevelly senna.

Senna is a stimulant laxative and is now used as the main ingredient in preparations for constipation, usually with carminatives to prevent griping. The active anthroquinones are liberated in the colon by the action of colonic bacteria. It may colour the urine a yellowish brown if the urine is acid, or red if alkaline.

It should not be taken by those with inflammatory colon diseases such as Crohn's disease or ulcerative colitis, nor for abdominal pain of unknown cause – which might be appendicitis.

It is used in homoeopathic medicine.

See Product Index for CONSTIPATION, PAIN (Oral) and URINARY TRACT.

## SEPIA

The dried, inky secretion of the cuttlefish, a cephalopod mollusc of the Sepiidae family, is used in homoeopathic medicine. Sepia is the Greek word for cuttlefish.

See Product Index for STRESS.

## SHARK    *various species* (Selachii)

Shark-liver oil is extracted from the liver of various species of shark.

This fixed oil contains a high level of vitamin A* and a little of vitamin D*.

Shark-liver oil is soothing and emollient and is used in haemorrhoidal preparations.

See Product Index for HAEMORRHOIDS.


## SHEPHERD'S PURSE    *Capsella bursa-pastoris* (Cruciferae)

This common plant grows wild throughout the world, taking its name from the shape of the seed cases. The whole dried plant contains flavonoids, plant acids and bases (histamine, tyramine, choline*).

Shepherd's Purse is astringent, diuretic and a urinary antiseptic. It is antiscorbutic, hypotensive and an emmenagogue, also haemostatic and stimulates the circulation, and thus is used to stop bleeding both internally and externally, for example excessive menstruation, haemorrhoids, blood in the urine, irritable bowel, nosebleeds and wounds. Shepherd's Purse is also used for cystitis and varicose veins.

See Product Index for PAIN (Oral) and URINARY TRACT.


## SILICON DIOXIDE Silica

This mineral, a major constituent of the earth's crust, occurs in many forms such as quartz, flint and, when in combination with other elements, as semi-precious stones like amethyst.

Colloidal silica is widely used in the manufacture of medicines, as a stabiliser in emulsions and as a suspending agent and thickener in suspensions, ointments and suppositories. In the production of tablets it is used as a granulating agent and lubricating agent, and because it adsorbs a large quantity of water without liquefying it is used as an anti-caking agent to prevent clogging of hygroscopic powders in the machinery during the manufacturing process. It is also used as a filler in tablet coatings.

It is listed in 'other ingredients' of many pharmaceutical products.

Silicon dioxide is called silicea when used in homoeopathic medicine. See Product Index for COLDS, HAY FEVER, PAIN (Oral) and SKIN.

**SILVER BIRCH** – see BIRCH

**SILYMARIN** – see MILK THISTLE

**SKULLCAP** – see SCULLCAP

**SKUNK CABBAGE**         *Symplocarpus foetidus* (Araceae)

A large deciduous perennial which is found in north-eastern USA, so named for the unpleasant smell that is produced when the plant is bruised.

The rhizome and roots contain resin, essential oil and serotonin. It is warming, sedative, analgesic and diaphoretic, also antispasmodic, diuretic, anticatarrhal and expectorant, and is used for bronchitis, asthma, irritating coughs, catarrh and hay fever.

See Product Index for COLDS.

**SLIPPERY ELM** Red Elm         *Ulmus fulva* (Ulmaceae)

A deciduous tree which grows in central and northern USA.

The inner bark is used, which contains mucilage.

Slippery elm is soothing, emollient, demulcent, nutritive, antitussive and expectorant, also diaphoretic, stomachic and vulnerary. Slippery elm is used as a mucilage to provide protection for inflammation or ulceration of the digestive tract and is often included in cough mixtures for its soothing properties. It can also be used as poultices for wounds, boils and other skin disorders where it soothes and draws.

See Product Index for HAEMORRHOIDS and INDIGESTION.

It is also sold as a food supplement.

**SLOE** – see BLACKTHORN

## SNAKE ROOT Senega          *Polygala senega* (Polygalaceae)

This perennial is native to the USA.

The roots contain phenolic acids and triterpene saponins, methyl salicylate* and sterols.

Snake root is diaphoretic, anti-inflammatory, diuretic, emetic and expectorant; it increases salivation and perspiration and is used for bronchitis, croup, catarrh and asthma, also for psoriasis and eczema.

See Product Index for COLDS.

## SODIUM – see MINERALS

## SODIUM BICARBONATE

Sodium bicarbonate neutralises the gastric acid, with liberation of carbon dioxide, and hence is used for dyspepsia. It makes mucous less viscous and so is used in nasal sprays and mouthwashes for the throat. It can be used as an eye lotion and as drops to soften ear wax. It makes the urine less acid and so can be used to treat cystitis. Large regular doses can be detrimental to those with hypertension due to the sodium content.

Sodium bicarbonate in solution can be used to treat bee stings (and in vinegar for wasps).

A dilute solution of sodium bicarbonate will remove iodine stains from the skin.

Sodium bicarbonate is used to make fizzy drinks and is an ingredient of baking powder, together with cream of tartar* or tartaric acid* – heating or wetting the mixture liberates carbon dioxide which, in baking, causes the dough to rise.

See Product Index for COLDS, CONSTIPATION, INDIGESTION and URINARY TRACT.

## SODIUM CHLORIDE Salt

It is an important mineral, essential to life, which regulates the amount of fluid entering the blood and the tissues and maintains the body's acid-alkali balance. Its role is controlled by the kidneys, an excess leading to fluid retention in the tissues and hypertension; too little causes hypotension. It is found in all body fluids, but is mainly present in the extracellular fluid. Excess salt is lost through sweating or in the urine; on a hot day people sweat more and lose a bit of salt in the sweat, but the body compensates for this by excreting less in the urine. People with high blood pressure should reduce their intake of salt, as the sodium in it increases blood pressure.

It is used in homoeopathy, where it is called natrum muriaticum or nat. mur.

See Product Index for COLDS, EYES, HAY FEVER, STRESS and VITAMINS, MINERALS & TONICS.

## SODIUM CITRATE

After absorption it is metabolised and acts similarly to sodium bicarbonate* in making the urine less acid. It is used in the treatment of inflammatory conditions of the bladder and cystitis. This is not suitable for those with high blood pressure because of the sodium it contains – they should use potassium citrate* instead.

## SODIUM SULPHATE Glauber's Salt

It is used as an osmotic laxative and as a diluent for food colours.

See Product Index for CONSTIPATION.

## SOYA                                    *Glycine soja* (Leguminosae)

The soya plant is grown as a crop throughout the world for its seeds (beans).

The oil, expressed from the seeds, contains linoleic acid, the most important of the polyunsaturated fatty acids. The beans themselves are also used as a food.

Soya is one of the few foods that contains all 22 amino acids. It is a rich source of lecithin*, which is a brain and nerve food, and protects the heart and arteries. Soya milk is a blend of water and the dehulled beans, which is easily digested and is used by those allergic to cow's milk. The emollient oil is used in the preparation of products for total parenteral nutrition for patients unable to eat food in the normal way. Soya bean sprouts are a rich source of vitamins* and minerals*.

Soya is a rich source of phytoestrogens (isoflavones), the major components being genistein and diazein. Soya isoflavones may be of help to menopausal women for hot flushes and other symptoms. However, it should not be taken by those who have, or have had in the past, an oestrogen-dependent (that is, oestrogen-receptor-positive) tumour such as breast, endometrial, cervical or ovarian cancer, as evidence of safety is not yet proven.

See Product Index for SKIN. It is sold as a food supplement.

## SPANISH FLY Cantharides          *Lytta vesicatoria* (Meloidae)

A golden-green European blister-beetle.

Cantharidin is extracted from dried beetles, especially from the wing cases and is rubefacient, counterirritant and vesicant.

It should not be taken orally or applied over large areas of the body owing to the risk of absorption through the skin.

Its use as an ingredient in cosmetics is prohibited by law in the United Kingdom. Spanish fly was formerly used as a blistering agent and was reputed to be aphrodisiac. It has been used in flexible collodion for the removal of warts and in the treatment of molluscum contagiosum.

Spanish fly is highly toxic and is no longer used in the UK medicinally except in homoeopathy, where it is known as cantharis.

See Product Index for FIRST AID and MOUTH.

## SPEARMINT                         *Mentha spicata* (Labiatae)

A common plant which grows in Britain, Europe, Asia, North Africa and the USA.

The leaves contain an essential oil, obtained by distillation, and flavonoids.

Spearmint resembles peppermint* in its action, being aromatic, antispasmodic, carminative and stimulant, and is used for digestive problems, dyspepsia, flatulence and abdominal cramps in the pharmaceutical, food and confectionery industries.

## SPIRULINA

A blue-green algae which has been promoted as a slimming aid.

It is sold as a food supplement.

## SPURGE Euphorbia          *Euphorbia hirta* (Euphorbiaceae)

A widespread weed. Spurge is derived from the Latin, *expurgare*, meaning 'to cleanse', or 'expurgate' – from the purgative properties of the juice.

The whole plant is used, containing terpenoids, flavonoids, choline* and gallic acid.

Spurge is antiseptic, expels phlegm and relieves spasms, hence its use for asthma and bronchitis, cough and catarrh. Spurge is also used for burns and warts. The sap from spurges growing in gardens can cause contact dermatitis.

See Product Index for COLDS.

## SQUALENE

This substance is found in certain fish oils, particularly shark-liver* oil and in certain vegetable oils – see olive* oil.

Squalene is a constituent of human sebum and so is used as an ingredient of ointments, as it increases skin permeability. It is also an intermediate of cholesterol metabolism and plays a key role in keeping the incidence of heart disease low in Mediterranean countries, where olive oil is a major component of the diet.

## SQUILL          *Drimia maritima* (Liliaceae)

A low-growing perennial, native to the Mediterranean region.

The bulbs contain flavonoids and cardiac glycosides.

Squill has a digitalis*-like effect on the heart; it is also antispasmodic, emetic, diuretic, stimulant, expectorant and antitussive, and so is used internally for bronchitis, bronchial asthma, whooping cough and oedema. Externally it is used in hair tonics for dandruff and seborrhoea.

See Product Index for COLDS.

## STARCH

It is a polysaccharide obtained from corn (maize), rice , wheat, potato or tapioca.

Starch is absorbent and so is included in dusting powders, either alone or with other ingredients, and also in some ointments. It is included in tablets as a disintegrating agent.

See Product Index for FIRST AID and SKIN.

It is also listed among 'other ingredients' of many products.


## STARFLOWER OIL – see GAMOLENIC ACID


## STARWORT – see FALSE UNICORN ROOT


## STAVESACRE        *Delphinium staphisagria* (Ranunculaceae)

The plant is native to the Mediterranean region. Staphisagria means 'wild raisin'.

The seeds, which contain alkaloids, are used as a lotion to kill parasites such as lice.

Stavesacre is too toxic for conventional internal use but is used in homoeopathic medicine.

See Product Index for NAUSEA & TRAVEL SICKNESS.


## STERCULIA Indian Tragacanth, Karaya        *Sterculia urens* (Sterculiaceae)

The gum of this tree is a complex polysaccharide, which also contains acetic acid*.

Sterculia is used as a bulk laxative. It has adhesive properties and so is used to assist in the fitting of ileostomy and colostomy appliances and in dental fixatives.

It is used in industry as a thickening and suspending agent in the manufacture of lotions and pastes.

See Product Index for CONSTIPATION.

**STINGING NETTLE** – see NETTLE

**STONE ROOT**  *Collinsonia canadensis* **(Labiatae)**

A perennial herb from Canada.

The rhizome is used which contains saponins, resin and essential oil.

Stone root is anti-inflammatory, diuretic, astringent and hepatic, and acts as a tonic to the digestive system and peripheral circulation. It dissolves kidney stones, hence its name.

As well as dissolving kidney and bladder stones, it is also used in herbal medicine for cystitis, diarrhoea, gastroenteritis and haemorrhoids.

See Product Index for CONSTIPATION.

**STORAX**  *Liquidambar orientalis* **(Hamamelidaceae)**

This deciduous tree is native to Asia Minor.

The balsam is obtained by beating the tree, this causes the balsam to be soaked up by the bark, which is then removed and boiled in water to release it. The balsam contains cinnamic acid, triterpenes and volatile oil.

Storax is antiseptic, anti-asthmatic, expectorant and stimulant, and its main use is as an ingredient of Friar's balsam*. It is also parasiticidal.

See Product Index for MOUTH.

**ST JOHN'S BREAD** – see CAROB

**ST JOHN'S WORT** Hypericum  *Hypericum perforatum* **(Hypericaceae)**

A plant which is native to Britain and Europe, with yellow flowers.

The leaves and flowers yield hypericin, hyperforin, flavonoids, phenols and essential oil. Hypericin is a red pigment, which can cause photosensitivity.

This herb is an aromatic, relaxing nervine, sedative and antidepressant, and is also astringent, antimicrobial, antiviral, anti-inflammatory and a cardiac tonic. It is also diuretic, expectorant, haemostatic and vulnery, and an emmenagogue. The flavonoids possess the analgesic and anti-inflammatory actions that are of benefit to those with neuralgia, sciatica and shingles. Hypericin and hyperforin influence the neurotransmitters in the brain and are responsible for the antidepressant activity, although all the substances in hypericum are needed to produce the overall balanced effect.

St John's wort has been used in recent years as an antidepressant. However it is only suitable for those with mild to moderate depression; those with moderate to severe depression should seek help from their doctor, and anyone already taking antidepressants prescribed by their doctor should not take this as well, as it may stop their prescribed antidepressant from working properly. If you think that St John's wort may help you, you should speak to your pharmacist first, as it interacts with a number of prescribed medicines (including the contraceptive pill) and so may not be appropriate for you to take.

Externally it is used for sores, bruises, burns, cramp and sprains – the caution above does not apply to creams, lotions and ointments.

It is used in both herbal and homoeopathic medicine.

Photosensitisation is a rare effect which can occur in some people.

It should not be used in pregnancy or while breast-feeding.

See Product Index for FIRST AID and PAIN (Oral) and (Topical). It is also sold as a food supplement.

## STRAMONIUM – see THORNAPPLE

## SULPHUR

A yellow non-metallic solid element found near volcanoes and in large underground deposits associated with oil. The old name for sulphur is brimstone.

Sulphur is a mild antiseptic which is keratolytic and antifungal, and has been widely used in lotions, creams and ointments for the treatment of skin disorders, such as acne.

A naturally occurring sulphur compound called methyl sulphonyl methane (MSM) originates in the ocean where microscopic plants called plankton release sulphur compounds, which in turn enter the food chain. This is one of the major building blocks of glucosaminoglycans, which are key structural components in cartilage, as well as hair and nails. MSM is sold as a food supplement for use with glucosamine* and chondroitin* in the treatment of arthritic conditions.

Sulphur is also used in homoeopathic medicine. See also MINERALS.

See Product Index for COLDS, CONSTIPATION, DIARRHOEA, HAEMORRHOIDS, HAIR & SCALP and SKIN.


## SUNDEW                    *Drosera rotundifolia* (Droseraceae)

This insectivorous plant grows throughout Europe on wet heaths and moors.

It contains quinones and flavonoids and is antitussive, anti-asthmatic, demulcent and antispasmodic, and is used for whooping cough, asthma and gastric complaints.

See Product Index for COLDS.


## SUNFLOWER                    *Helianthus annus* (Compositae)

The sunflower is dedicated to Helios, the Greek sun god.

Widely grown throughout the world, they grow up to three metres high with large bright-yellow flowers. The seeds form in the centre of the flower. When ripe, they are harvested.

The fixed oil is expressed from the fruits (seeds), which are rich in minerals* and vitamins* B and E. The oil is rich in gamolenic acid*, an omega-6 triglyceride.

Sunflower oil is nutritive, lowers cholesterol, is antitussive and soothes inflamed tissues.

The seeds are eaten to strengthen muscles and improve the performance of athletes.

The oil is used in cooking, in place of olive* oil and in margarine.

See Product Index for FIRST AID and PAIN (Oral).

## SWAMP TEA TREE – see CAJUPUT

## SWEET FLAG Calamus            *Acorus calamus* (Araceae)

The plant grows on river banks and marshy places in America and Europe.

The dried rhizome and root are used; they contain a bitter, aromatic, volatile oil containing terpenes.

Sweet flag is used as a bitter carminative, which is antispasmodic, and also to flavour alcoholic beverages. The oil is used in perfumery.

This herb should not be used in pregnancy or while breast-feeding.

See Product Index for INDIGESTION.

## SWEET ORANGE OIL – see ORANGE OIL

## SWEET ROOT – see LIQUORICE

## SURGICAL SPIRIT

It contains castor* oil, diethyl phalate, methyl salicylate* and industrial methylated spirit .

It is applied externally for its astringent action. It should not be applied to mucous membranes or broken skin. It should not be taken internally because of the methyl alcohol it contains.

## TALC

A purified, native, hydrated magnesium silicate, which may contain a small amount of aluminium sulphate. It needs to be sterilised before use in manufacture, due to bacterial contamination.

Purified talc is used in massage and as a dusting powder to allay irritation and prevent chafing. It is usually mixed with starch* and zinc oxide* for these purposes. It is used as a lubricant in making tablets and to clarify liquids.

See Product Index for SKIN.

## TARAXACUM – see DANDELION

## TARTAR, CREAM OF Potassium Acid Tartrate

It is used as a purgative. It also has a mild diuretic action.

Cream of tartar, or tartaric acid*, is used as an ingredient of baking powder, together with sodium bicarbonate*.

## TARTARIC ACID

It is used in the preparation of effervescent powders, granules and tablets; it is used as an ingredient of cooling drinks and baking powder, and as a purgative.

## TEA                    *Camellia sinensis* (Theaceae)

This shrub is cultivated in China, Sri Lanka, Indonesia and elsewhere.

Green tea is produced in China and Japan, black tea in India, Sri Lanka and Kenya.

The leafbuds and very young leaves contain caffeine*, with smaller amounts of other xanthines* such as theophylline* and theobromine. Tea also contains tannins, flavonoids (including quercetin*) and flavour compounds.

It is a stimulant and a diuretic due to the caffeine, and astringent due to the tannins.

It is useful in diarrhoea and is drunk throughout the world for its refreshing, stimulating and mildy analgesic effects.

## TEA TREE          *Melaleuca alternifolia* (Myrtaceae)

An evergreen tree from Australia.

It contains a volatile oil, obtained by steam distillation of the foliage and terminal branches, which contains terpenes, terpineol* and cineole, which is also found in eucalyptus*. This oil is also called melaleuca oil.

The non-irritating, non-poisonous oil is antiseptic, bactericidal, antiviral and antifungal. It stimulates the immune system.

Tea tree oil should not be taken internally and should only be used neat for application to verrucas and warts. For all others uses it should be diluted with a carrier oil, when it can be applied for athlete's foot, insect bites, acne, cold sores and thrush. It can also be used for pimples, boils and infected wounds.

The essential oil is used in aromatherapy.

See Product Index for FIRST AID and SKIN.


## TERPINEOL

A constituent of some essential oils, including cardamom*, orange* and tea tree* oils.

It has antibacterial and solvent properties and is used as a flavouring agent.

See Product Index for COLDS, EARS, PAIN (Topical) and SKIN.


## THEOPHYLLINE

An alkaloid found in some plants such as cocoa* and coffee* – a xanthine*.

Theophylline relaxes smooth muscle and relieves bronchspasm; it stimulates the heart and respiration and is diuretic.

It is used in the treatment of asthma and bronchitis.

See Product Index for COLDS.


## THIAMINE – see VITAMIN B1

## THORNAPPLE Stramonium

*Datura stramonium*
(Solanaceae)

A bushy annual native to North and South America.

The dried leaves, flowering tops and seeds contain alkaloids, including hyoscyamine, with smaller amounts of hyoscine* and atropine*. The seeds also contain coumarins, tannins and a fixed oil.

Thornapple is a narcotic nerve sedative which is antispasmodic, anti-asthmatic, analgesic, and encourages healing. In herbal medicine it is used for treating asthma and for excessive salivation as in Parkinson's disease. Externally it is used for severe neuralgia.

It is used in homoeopathic medicine.

It should not be used in pregnancy, while breast-feeding, nor with heart failure or prostatitis.

## THYME Common, Garden

*Thymus vulgaris* (Labiatae)

Thyme is indigenous to the Mediterranean region and is widely cult-ivated. Its name is from the Greek, meaning 'courage' (it was used by soldiers), or 'sacrifice', as it was originally used as an incense in the temples.

The whole plant contains a volatile oil (thymol*), tannins, gum and flavonoids.

This herb is antiseptic, antibiotic, antifungal, antiviral, an immune stimulant, expectorant, antitussive and antioxidant, a diaphoretic febrifuge, carminative, stomachic, tonic, and diuretic, and is also a mild sedative. Thyme is rubefacient and insect repellent.

Thyme has been used as an ingredient in cough linctuses for dry coughs, whooping cough, bronchitis, bronchial catarrh and sinusitis, and relieves bronchial spasm and reduces the viscosity of the mucus. It is used as a mouthwash for mouth ulcers and gingivitis, and as a gargle for sore throat. It is used externally in liniments as a rubefacient and counterirritant. The oil is used in aromatherapy.

It should be avoided in pregnancy.

See Product Index for COLDS, PAIN (Topical) and SKIN.

## THYMOL

The volatile oil extracted from thyme* consists mainly of thymol, which is used as an antiseptic, deodorant, mouthwash and gargle. Thymol is also found in arnica*, calumba* and damiana*. It is used in dentistry to prepare cavities for filling and with zinc oxide* as a protective cap for the dentine. It is used in inhalants with other volatile oils for coughs, colds and respiratory disorders.

See Product Index for COLDS and SKIN.

## TILIA – see LIME

## TINNEVELLY SENNA – see SENNA

## TOLU                    *Myroxylon balsamum* (Leguminosae)

This evergreen tree is native to South America and is also cultivated in the West Indies. A balsam is obtained by incising the trunk of the tree which contains triterpenoids, benzoic acid* and cinnamic acid.

Tolu is a stimulating expectorant and antiseptic which is used in the preparation of cough mixtures and is an ingredient of Friar's balsam. It is also used in the preparation of throat lozenges and pastilles. Tolu Syrup BP is now based on cinnamic acid.

See Product Index for COLDS.

## TRAGACANTH              *Astralagus gummifer* (Leguminosae)

This shrub grows in the Middle East, especially Turkey and Syria; the name is from the Greek, *tragos*, for goat thorn.

Tragacanth is the dried, gummy exudate which flows naturally or is obtained by incision of the branches of the shrub and which contains a water-soluble polysaccharide, tragacanthin, and an insoluble poly-saccharide, bassorin. It also contains starch*, cellulose, invert sugar and acetic acid*. It is demulcent, mucilaginous, emollient and laxative; it stimulates the immune system. Tragacanth is mainly used as a stabilising and thickening agent in the pharmaceutical and food industries; it has been used in lozenges for its demulcent properties and as a bulk laxative.

## TREACLE

Treacle is derived from the Greek, *theriake*, meaning 'antidote for the bite of wild beasts'. In ancient times the name was used for several sorts of antidote, but was applied mainly to Venice treacle (theriaca androchi), a compound of some 64 drugs in honey. Today, however, treacle refers to the uncrystallisable residue from sugar-refining.

See Product Index for COLDS and SKIN.

## TURMERIC *Curcuma longa* (Zingiberaceae)

This plant comes from southern Asia and is now cultivated in other tropical countries. The name is from the Latin, *terra merita*, meaning 'deserving earth', which is appropriate for a plant that grows underground and so has its essence from the earth.

The rhizome contains curcuminoids, including curcumin, a powerful antioxidant the main function of which is to repair and protect the liver. It also contains volatile oil.

Although seldom used medicinally, it is anti-inflammatory, antibilious, being a hepatic cholagogue, as well as being anticholesterol. It is antioxidant, antimicrobial and haemostatic.

Turmeric is important in the preparation of curry powders and as a natural colouring agent in foodstuffs.

See Product Index for INDIGESTION.

## TURPENTINE various species including *Pinus palustris* (Pinaceae)

Pine trees are evergreen and coniferous and grow in many parts of the world.

An oleo-resin is obtained as an exudate from the tree, and turpentine oil is obtained from this by distillation and rectification. It consists mainly of pinenes and some terpenes.

Turpentine oil is used externally as a rubefacient and counterirritant. It is to be found in liniments for rheumatic pain and stiffness.

See Product Index for COLDS, EARS and PAIN (Oral).

## TWITCH – see COUCHGRASS

# U

**ULMARIA** – see MEADOWSWEET

## UREA

Originally obtained from urine but now produced synthetically.

Urea is an osmotic diuretic, which is anaesthetic, bactericidal and keratolytic.

It is used in creams for the treatment of ichthyosis and hyperkeratotic skin disorders. Its effect is probably dependent on increased hydration, although it may be irritant to sensitive skin.

See Product Index for SKIN.

**URTICA** – see NETTLE

**UVA URSI** – see BEARBERRY

## VALERIAN                    *Valeriana officinalis* (Valerianaceae)

This perennial is native to Europe and Asia; it is naturalised in the USA. The name, valerian is from the Latin, *valere*, 'to be healthy'.

The rhizomes and roots contain alkaloids, iridoids known as valepotriates, organic acids and essential oil. Valerian also contains choline*, flavonoids, sterols and tannins.

It acts as a natural relaxant to the nervous system. Valerenic acid inhibits breakdown of GABA (gamma-aminobutyric acid), a neurotransmitter in the brain. This helps to decrease activity in the brain, which explains why valerian is sedative, hypnotic and relaxant; it is aromatic, expectorant, carminative and is an emmenagogue, antigout and hypotensive. It relaxes spasms, relieves pain and improves the digestion. Valerian is a stimulant nervine and is also antidepressant.

It is used for stress, anxiety and sleeplessness. It has been shown to improve the quality of sleep, reduce the time taken to fall asleep and does not cause somnolence the following morning. It is also used for tension headaches and migraine, menstrual, muscle and intestinal cramps, and externally it is used for eczema and minor injuries.

The oil is used in perfumery.

It should not be taken by those with liver problems, or during pregnancy or while breast-feeding.

See Product Index for COLDS, CONSTIPATION, INDIGESTION, PAIN (Oral), SLEEP and STRESS.

## VEGETABLE CHARCOAL – see CHARCOAL

## VERVAIN                    *Verbena officinalis* (Verbenaceae)

This plant grows throughout Europe, especially in the south.

The whole plant is used, which contains iridoids, choline*, flavonoids and volatile oil.

A bitter, aromatic, astringent, diaphoretic, diuretic herb, which is antispasmodic, anti-inflammatory, analgesic, an emmenagogue, emetic and haemostatic; it is a tonic sedative nervine which calms the nerves, improves liver and gall bladder function and stimulates the uterus. It also has antidepressant and anticonvulsant properties.

Vervain is used for nervous exhaustion and depression, post-viral fatigue syndrome and ME (myalgic encephalomyelitis), also for congested liver and gall bladder problems, to promote milk production in nursing mothers, and in asthma and migraine.

It should not be taken in pregnancy.

See Product Index for PAIN (Oral), SLEEP and STRESS.


## VINCA ALKALOIDS – see PERIWINKLE


## VITAMINS

Vitamins are essential to the normal-functioning of the body and, with the exception of niacin and vitamin D, we cannot manufacture them ourselves. We obtain them in the food we eat. There are 13 vitamins: A, C, D, E, K and B12 – cyanocobalamin, and seven which are the B-complex vitamins – B1 (thiamine), B2 (riboflavin), B3 (niacin), B5 (pantothenic acid), B6 (pyridoxine), folic acid and biotin (also known as vitamin H).

Vitamins A, D, E and K are fat-soluble. Excess intake may be harmful as the body stores them in the fatty tissues.

Vitamins B12, the B complex and C are water-soluble. The body can only store a limited amount; any excess is excreted in the urine.

Other substances that cannot strictly be considered to be vitamins, although they are an essential factor in human nutrition, are choline and inositol. Bioflavonoids used to be referred to as vitamin P – see quercetin*.

**Vitamin A**
**(retinol)** – comes from animal sources such as liver, kidney and dairy products. Vitamin A is essential for growth and for the development and maintenance of epithelial tissue and for vision. It is an antioxidant, like vitamins C and E, which means it neutralises free radicals; free radicals may damage tissues in rheumatoid arthritis, thrombosis, heart failure, cancer and when the immune system is weakened.

Women who are pregnant or breast-feeding should avoid high levels of vitamin A because of possible birth defects. This is why they are advised to not to eat liver, which contains high levels, during pregnancy.

**Beta-carotene** – a precursor of vitamin A is found in plant sources such as red, orange or yellow fruit and vegetables, such as apricots, peaches, tomatoes, carrots and peppers; it is converted to vitamin A by the liver.

**Vitamin B1**
**(thiamine)** – is found in liver, pork, wholegrain cereals, pulses, nuts, milk and bread. It is essential for the metabolism of carbohydrates, fat and alcohol into energy. It is required for growth and is important for the heart and nervous system.

**Vitamin B2**
**(riboflavin)** – is found in milk, eggs, liver, fish and green vegetables. It is needed for growth and development, also for healthy skin, hair and nerves.

**Vitamin B3**
**(niacin=** – found in oily fish, meat, whole cereals and nuts.
**nicotinic acid,** It is needed for the nervous system, skin and
**is converted** energy production from food.
**to active form**
**nicotinamide)**

**Vitamin B5**
**(pantothenic** – is found in meat, dairy products and eggs. It is
**acid)** needed for metabolism of carbohydrates and fats to provide energy, for healthy hair and skin.

**Vitamin B6**
(pyridoxine)
– is found in fish, whole cereals and bread and is needed for healthy blood vessels and nervous system. Those taking anticonvulsants or levadopa should avoid supplements containing pyridoxine.

**Vitamin B12**
(cobalamin)
– is found in foods of animal origin and is essential for production of red blood cells and is fundamental to growth. Vegetarians who exclude dairy products and vegans need to supplement their diet with this vitamin.

**Folic acid**
– is found in liver, pulses, green vegetables, wheatgerm, wholemeal bread and yeast extract. Folic acid is vital in the early stages of pregnancy – a dose of 400 micrograms daily should be taken by women in the months before and during the first part of pregnancy as this vitamin helps prevent spinabifida in the developing baby. Some women on other medication (such as epileptics), may need to take a much higher dose at this time which will be prescribed by their doctor. Recent work suggests a higher incidence of twins for women taking folic acid supplements. It is needed by everyone for the production of red blood cells.

**Biotin**
(sometimes called vitamin H)
– is found in wholegrain cereals, pulses, nuts and eggs. It is needed for a healthy skin and for the metabolism of proteins and fats.

**Vitamin C**
(ascorbic acid)
– is found in fruit, especially citrus fruit, and vegetables. It is needed for healthy gums, to heal wounds and for a healthy immune system. It is an antioxidant, like vitamins A and E. High doses can interfere with glucose-monitoring tests and so should be avoided by diabetics who use these tests.

| | |
|---|---|
| **Vitamin D** (calciferol) | – is found in oily fish and their oils, also in eggs, butter and milk. The body can produce vitamin D by the action of sunlight on the skin. It is essential to the absorption of calcium from the diet, for strong bones and teeth, and in the treatment of osteoporosis – see calcium carbonate*. |
| **Vitamin E** | – is found in vegetable oils, wholegrain cereals, nuts, eggs and some vegetables. Like vitamin A and C it is an antioxidant. |
| **Vitamin K** | – is found in wholegrain cereals, pulses and nuts. It is essential to blood clotting, so much so that every newborn baby is given an injection of it soon after birth. Those taking anticoagulants should not take supplements containing vitamin K. |

See Product Index for VITAMINS, MINERALS & TONICS.

They are also sold as food supplements.

## WAHOO Euonymus

*Euonymus atropurpureus*
**(Celastraceae)**

This is a large deciduous shrubby tree which grows in eastern and central USA and Canada. Wahoo is a Dakota Indian word, meaning arrow wood.

The bark from the stem and roots contain alkaloids, sterols, tannins and cardenolides.

Wahoo is a stimulant to the liver and gall bladder, and is diuretic, laxative and increases cardiac tone. It is taken for constipation and problems caused by liver and gall bladder.

It should not be taken in pregnancy or whilst breast-feeding.

See Product Index for INDIGESTION.

## WATERCRESS

*Nasturtium officinalis* (Cruciferae)

An aquatic perennial plant found in Europe and Central Asia.

The leaves are rich in iron, phophorus, potassium, manganese, iodine*, sulphur* and folic acid – see also minerals* and vitamins*.

Watercress is an immune stimulant, antioxidant and antiscorbutic, expectorant and diuretic, and improves the digestion and enriches the blood.

Traditionally taken as a spring tonic, the leaves can be added to salads.

It is used for catarrh, bronchitis, coughs, and for anaemia, debility and rheumatism.

See Product Index for PAIN (Oral) and URINARY TRACT.

## WAX MYRTLE – see BAYBERRY

## WHITE BRYONY – see BRYONY, WHITE

## WHITE HOREHOUND – see HOREHOUND

## WHITE WALNUT – see BUTTERNUT

## WILD CARROT  *Daucus carota* (Umbelliferae)

This is the wild form of the garden carrot and is found in Europe, North Africa and Asia.

The whole plant yields an alkaloid (daucine), flavonoids and a volatile oil.

Wild carrot is diuretic, antispasmodic, carminative and a rich source of beta-carotene (precursor of vitamin A*); it resolves stones of the kidney and bladder, and so is used for urinary stones, gout and cystitis; and also for menstrual problems, menopausal hot flushes, flatulent indigestion and oedema. The beta-carotene helps improve vision, especially at night.

The oil is used in the preparation of anti-wrinkle creams.

See Product Index for Pain (Oral) and URINARY TRACT.


## WILD INDIGO  *Baptisia tinctoria* (Leguminosae)

This perennial plant grows in Canada and the USA.

The dried roots contain flavonoids, coumarins, isoflavones and a bitter principle, baptisin.

Wild indigo is a bitter, alternative, antiseptic herb that is anticatarrhal, decongestant, hepatic, laxative and emetic; it stimulates the immune system, lowers fever and is antimicrobial, antibiotic, antifungal and antiviral. It is used for throat and chest infections, and externally for boils, ulcers, sore nipples and vaginitis.

See Product Index for FIRST AID and VITAMINS, MINERALS & TONICS.


## WILD LETTUCE  *Lactuca virosa* (Compositae)

The wild lettuce is similar to garden lettuce and is indigenous to central and southern Europe and northern Asia.

The leaves and latex contain flavonoids, coumarins, lactucin and hyoscyamine.

Wild Lettuce is a bitter, sedative nerve relaxant, and is a diaphoretic, diuretic, narcotic, mild hypnotic and also a mild analgesic. It is anti-gout, antispasmodic, antitussive and expectorant.

It is used for anxiety, stress and insomnia, and for coughs, bronchitis and rheumatic pain.

See Product Index for COLDS, PAIN (Oral) and SLEEP.

## WILD PANSY Heartsease    *Viola tricolor* (Violaceae)

This plant is widely distributed throughout temperate regions of the world.

The whole plant is used, which contains flavonoids, saponins, mucilage and gum. The flavonoids stabilise capillary membranes, which is important in inflammatory skin conditions. The saponins soothe inflamed areas of skin and improve the blood flow to the kidneys, so increasing the elimination of toxins.

Wild pansy is a bitter–sweet, diuretic, expectorant, laxative herb, which lowers fever and relieves pain, reduces inflammation, cleanses toxins and promotes healing.

Internally it is used for rheumatism, bronchitis, cough, skin (especially weeping eczema) and urinary complaints, also for capillary fragility, and externally for skin complaints and varicose ulcers.

See Product Index for SKIN.

## WILD ROSE – see ROSE

## WILD STRAWBERRY    *Fragaria vesca* (Rosaceae)

It is widely cultivated.

The leaves are used and the fruit is eaten. The leaves contain tropane alkaloids, mainly hyoscyamine and hyoscine* and some atropine* – see Belladonna.

Wild strawberry is spasmolytic, anti-anaemic, anti-asthmatic and anticholinergic, and so causes dryness of the mouth. It is also haemostatic, astringent, diuretic and laxative, and is used for colitis, irritable bowel, kidney and bladder gravel and gallstones.

See Product Index for INDIGESTION, PAIN (Oral) and STRESS.

## WILD YAM Colic Root, Rheumatism Root
### *Dioscorea villosa* (Dioscoriaceae)

This perennial climber is common in eastern and central USA and some tropical countries. The Latin name is a tribute to the Greek physician and botanist, Dioscorides.

The root, which has been used in China for more than 2,000 years, contains steroidal saponins. Many species of *Dioscorea* are used as sources of saponins for the preparation of steroids for the pharmaceutical industry. For some years prior to 1970 the Mexican Yam was the sole source for production of the contraceptive pill, before the industry was able to produce the starting material synthetically.

Wild Yam is analgesic, anti-asthmatic, anti-inflammatory and antispasmodic. It is also diuretic, stomachic and antibilious, acting on the liver and gall bladder, a nervine and antipruritic. As its common names suggest, it is used for rheumatism and colic, also for painful periods and cramps.

It should not be used in pregnancy and should not be taken by those who have, or have had in the past, an oestrogen-dependent (that is oestrogen-receptor-positive) tumour such as breast, endometrial, cervical or ovarian cancer, as evidence of safety is not yet proven.

It is promoted as a natural form of hormone replacement therapy (HRT) and is sold as a food supplement.

## WILLOW White Willow
### *Salix alba* (Salicaceae)

The willow tree is indigenous to Britain, central and southern Europe.

The dried bark contains flavonoids, tannins, and phenolic glycosides. It contains salicylic acid* and has been used for thousands of years for fevers and as a pain-killer: it can be regarded as the natural form and origin of the modern aspirin. (It is only about a hundred years ago that acetylsalicylic acid [aspirin] was first synthesised.)

Willow relieves pain, lowers fever and reduces inflammation; it is also antiseptic, astringent, tonic, antirheumatic and antigout. It is used to relieve the pain and inflammation of rheumatism, gout and arthritis, for neuralgia, headache and feverish illnesses. See Product Index for INDIGESTION and PAIN (Oral).

It is also sold as a food supplement.

## WINTERGREEN  *Gaultheria procumbens* (Ericaceae)

This creeping shrublet is native to North America and Canada.

The leaves contain an oil which is almost completely composed of methyl salicylate. It is also a source of salicin, and other phenolic compounds.

Methyl salicylate has a similar effect to aspirin, being anti-inflammatory; it is also a good antiseptic, rubefacient and counterirritant, and is diuretic and expectorant. It is an astringent, stimulant tonic which is antirheumatic.

Oil of wintergreen is used, mainly externally, for rheumatoid arthritis, inflammation of joints, muscles and sprains, and for lumbago, backache and neuralgia. It is also used for chilblains and in inhalations for symptomatic relief of upper respiratory disorders.

Absorption through the skin can occur following excessive application so caution should be taken by those taking anticoagulants, such as warfarin.

It should not be given to those who are sensitive to aspirin.

See Product Index for COLDS, FIRST AID, HAIR & SCALP, PAIN (Topical) and SKIN.

## WITCH HAZEL  *Hamamelis virginiana* (Hamamelidaceae)

A deciduous shrub or small tree, indigenous to North America and Canada. The common name refers to the occult powers attributed to the plant, whose hazel-like branches were used as divining rods in times past in the search for water or gold.

The bark and leaves contain tannins, flavonoids, saponins, gallic acid and a trace of volatile oil.

Witch hazel is cooling, cleansing and astringent, haemostatic, anti-inflammatory, antifungal, healing, antipruritic and vulnerary. It is used for bruising, sprains and varicose veins, haemorrhoids, sore nipples, nosebleeds and chilblains and also for conjunctivitis and tired eyes. It is no longer used internally.

It is used in herbal and homoeopathic medicine. See Product Index for EYES, FIRST AID, HAEMORRHOIDS, HAIR & SCALP, and SKIN.

**WOLFSBANE** – see ACONITE and ARNICA

## WOOL ALCOHOLS

It is obtained by saponification of wool fat – see lanolin* – and is used in the preparation of emulsions and ointments.

See Product Index for FIRST AID, PAIN (Topical) and SKIN.

**WOOLFAT** – see LANOLIN

## XANTHAN GUM

This is produced by a pure culture fermentation of a carbohydrate with *Xanthomonas campestris*, which is then purified.

It is used in pharmaceutical manufacture and in the food industry as an emulsifying, suspending, stabilising and thickening agent.

## XANTHINES

Xanthines are alkaloids, to be found in chocolate, cocoa*, coffee*, kola*, maté* and tea*.

The main xanthine present is caffeine*, but some also contain theophylline* and theobromine. See individual entries for further information.

Xanthines are central nervous system stimulants and are also diuretic.

## YARROW Milfoil, Achillea

*Achillea millefolium*
(Compositea)

A plant native to Eurasia and found in most temperate parts of the world. Yarrow, or Achillea, got its name because it was used by Achilles to heal his warriors in the Trojan War; an old country name was soldier's woundwort, for its ability to staunch blood flow.

The dried flowering tops are used. The herb contains a volatile oil, alkaloids, a bitter principle (ivain), and various tannins.

Yarrow has been used for a great variety of medicinal purposes, in herbal and homoeopathic medicine, being astringent, anti-inflammatory, antirheumatic, antigout, antispasmodic, antipyretic, carminative, bitter and haemostatic. It is also antimicrobial, anti-catarrhal, a diaphoretic febrifuge, a cardiac tonic and hypotensive.

Today it is used to treat rheumatism, indigestion, colds, catarrh, fevers and hypertension.

It is used in herbal and homoeopathic medicine.

It can cause contact dermatitis and photosensitivity.

See Product Index for COLDS, CONSTIPATION, INDIGESTION , PAIN (Oral) and STRESS. It is also sold as a food supplement.

## YEAST Brewer's Yeast

*Saccharomyces species*
(Saccharomycetaceae)

It is a rich source of vitamins* of the B group, containing thiamine, nicotinic acid, riboflavine, pyridoxine, pantothenic acid, biotin, folic acid, cyanocobalamin, aminobenzoic acid, inositol* and chromium (see minerals*).

Yeast is used in preparations for haemorrhoids and some preparations intended to restore the normal gastrointestinal flora, and as a dietary supplement.

It is also used in baking and brewing.

See Product Index for HAEMORRHOIDS, INDIGESTION, PAIN (Oral) and SLEEP.

## YELLOW DOCK – see DOCK

## YELLOW ROOT – see GOLDEN SEAL

## YEW                                   *Taxus brevifolia* (Taxaceae)

This large evergreen tree, also used as hedging, is grown as an ornamental in Britain, America and other parts of the world.

The leaves and bark, provided from the hedge clippings of stately homes from their ornamental gardens and mazes, contain taxanes which are extracted by the pharmaceutical industry in the preparation of drugs for use in the treatment of cancer of the lungs, breasts and ovaries. Paclitaxel was formerly called taxol, but Taxol is now a brand name used by the manufacturer.

**ZANTHOXYLUM** – see PRICKLY ASH

**ZINC** – see MINERALS

## ZINC OXIDE

It occurs naturally as zincite.

It is a mild astringent which is soothing and protective and is used in a wide variety of creams, pastes and ointments for the treatment of skin conditions such as eczema, and also in medicated bandages, liniments and lotions.

See Product Index for FIRST AID, HAEMORRHOIDS and SKIN.

# Part 2

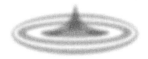

The Product Index of
Licensed Medicines

Most, if not all, of the products listed are available from your local pharmacy. If they do not normally stock the item you want, it can be ordered from the pharmaceutical wholesaler very quickly and should be ready for collection from the pharmacy in the next day or so.

Some manufacturers also have a mail-order service available to the general public. Their addresses are listed in Part 3 of this book

## Colds, Coughs, Influenza, Catarrh and Sore Throats

There is no cure for the common cold or influenza; however there are many medicines and remedies available that can offer some degree of relief from the symptoms, although those who suffer with long-term chest conditions, such as bronchitis or emphysema, should see their doctor rather than trying to treat themselves. The elderly and other at-risk groups should ensure they receive an annual influenza vaccination.

Some of the listed products should not be taken in pregnancy or whilst breast-feeding; some are not suitable for children. Ask your pharmacist for advice on suitability.

Some cough and cold remedies may not be suitable for people with high blood pressure, thyroid problems, coronary heart disease, diabetes, glaucoma, enlarged prostate or those taking monoamine oxidase inhibitors (MAOIs). Any prescribed medication should be mentioned to your pharmacist at the time of purchase so that an appropriate product can be chosen. Also diabetics should be aware of the high sugar content of some cough mixtures – sugar-free versions are available.

| Products | Uses | Ingredients |
|---|---|---|

## Herbal

| Products | Uses | Ingredients |
|---|---|---|
| Bioforce<br>– Echinaforce<br>  Drops and Tablets | relief of colds, influenza-type infections and similar upper-respiratory-tract conditions | echinacea |
| – Lobelia Compound | for coughs, blocked sinuses, catarrh | lobelia, squill, gum ammon |
| Dorwest Garlic and Fenugreek Tablets | coughs, colds, catarrh and rhinitis | fenugreek and garlic |
| Gerard House<br>– Catarrh-eeze | for effective relief of catarrh | horehound, elecampne, yarrow |
| – Echinacea & Garlic | for colds and influenza | echinacea, garlic |
| Hactos Cough Mixture | coughs, colds, catarrh | capsicum, peppermint, anise, clove |
| Herbal Concepts<br>– Asthma and<br>  Catarrh Relief | temporary relief of bronchial asthma and catarrh | ipecacuanha, lobelia, horehound and liquorice |
| – Hay Fever and<br>  Sinus Relief | hay fever, catarrh and sinus congestion | echinacea, elder flower, garlic |
| Hofels<br>– Garlic and Parsley | coughs and colds | garlic |
| – Garlic One-a-day | coughs and colds | garlic |
| HRI Garlic Tablets | catarrh and rhinitis | garlic |
| Lane's<br>– Herbelix Specific<br>  Mixture | catarrh, hay fever, rhinitis, mucous congestion,head cold | lobelia, tolu, sodium bicarbonate |
| – Honey and Molasses<br>  Mixture | coughs, colds, sore throat | ipecacuanha, horehound, squill |
| – Sinotar Tablets | blocked sinuses and catarrh | marshmallow, echinacea elder flower |
| Lusty's Garlic Perles | catarrh, rhinitis, common cold | garlic |

C

| Products | Uses | Ingredients |
|---|---|---|
| Modern Herbals | | |
| – Cold and Catarrh Tablets | blocked sinuses and catarrh | marshmallow, echinacea, elder flower |
| – Cough Mixture | coughs, colds, hoarseness, sore throats and catarrh | ipecacuanha, horehound, squill |
| – Cold and Congestion Syrup | catarrh, hay fever, rhinitis, mucous congestion and head cold | lobelia, tolu and sodium bicarbonate |
| Phytocold | assists resistance to common cold infections of nose, throat and head | echinacea |
| Potter's | | |
| – Antibron | coughs | lobelia, coltsfoot, euphorbia, pleurisy root, snake root, wild lettuce |
| – Antifect | catarrh, rhinitis, nasal congestion | garlic, garlic oil, echinacea |
| – Balm of Gilead | coughs | balm of gilead, squill, lobelia and lungwort |
| – Catarrh Mixture | catarrh of the nose and throat | boneset, blue flag, burdock, hyssop, capsicum |
| – Chest Mixture | coughs and catarrh | horehound, pleurisy root, snake root, lobelia, squill |
| – Echinacea Elixir | catarrh of the nose and throat, minor skin conditions, immunostimulant | echinacea, wild indigo, fumitory |
| – EP&C Essence | colds, chills, sore throats | bayberry, hemlock spruce elder flower, peppermint oil |
| – Garlic | colds, coughs, rhinitis | garlic and garlic oil |
| – Horehound and Aniseed Cough Mixture | coughs | pleurisy root, elecampne, horehound, skunk cabbage, lobelia |
| – Life Drops | influenza, colds, chills, and sore throat | capsicum, elder flower, peppermint oil |
| – Lightning Cough Remedy | for coughs | liquorice, aniseeed |
| – Peerless Composition Essence | colds and chills | oak bark, hemlock spruce, poplar, prickly ash, bayberry |

193

| Products | Uses | Ingredients |
|---|---|---|
| – Vegetable Cough Remover | coughs, wheezing, colds, catarrh | capsicum, black cohosh, lobelia, ipecacuanha, pleurisy root, scullcap, skunk cabbage, valerian, elecampne, horehound, hyssop, aniseed, liquorice |
| Revitonil | colds and upper respiratory tract infections | liquorice, eucalyptus, aniseed, fennel, peppermint, cloves |
| Ricola Lozenges | stuffy nose, sore throat, cough | menthol, peppermint oil |
| Weleda Herb and Honey Cough Elixir | dry and irritating coughs | marshmallow, elder, horehound, iceland moss, aniseed, thyme, honey, glycerol, citric acid |

## Homoeopathic

| | | |
|---|---|---|
| aconite | for dry, irritating cough, beginnings of cold and flu' | aconite |
| allium cepa | for cold with sneezing, watery eyes and nasal discharge | onion |
| apis mel | for sore throat: swollen, painful, bright red | honey-bee |
| arsen alb | for wheezy, burning sensation in chest, streaming eyes and nose | arsenic trioxide |
| belladonna | for dry, tickly, barking cough, high temperature and fever, face and throat hot, swallowing painful | belladonna |
| bryonia | for hard dry cough with headache, dry mouth and throat, catarrh on chest which feels tight | bryony |
| calc carb | for tickly cough with yellow sputum | calcium carbonate |
| calc fluor | for sore throat pain, worse at night and from drinks, and yellow/green catarrh, worst after rest | calcium fluoride |
| drosera | for persistent, irritating cough from deep in chest | sundew |

**C**

| Products | Uses | Ingredients |
|---|---|---|
| euphrasia | for pronounced sneezing and watery eyes and catarrh | eyebright |
| ferrum phos | for feverishness, stuffiness and sneezing | iron phosphate |
| gelsemium | for hot and cold shivering flu' symptoms, sore throat | gelsemium |
| hepar sulph | for hoarse cough with sore throat | calcium sulphide |
| kali bich | for coughs with stringy phlegm, yellow discharge with sore throat | potassium bichromate |
| nat mur | for cough with pain in head, frequent sneezing, dripping nose | sodium chloride |
| nux vom | for dry, tearing, spasmodic cough with retching, and colds with much sneezing, sore throat | nux vomica |
| phosphorus | for violent hard dry cough with yellow sputum | phosphoric acid |
| pulsatilla | for cough dry in morning, loose at night, catarrh worse at night | pasque flower |
| silicea | for sinusitis and headaches, slow onset and recovery | silicon dioxide |
| Nelson's | | |
| – Coldenza | influenza and influenza-like colds | gelsemium |
| – Sootha Tablets | coughs | white bryony |
| – Sootha Syrup | coughs | white bryony, honey, lemon |
| New Era Tissue Salts: | | |
| – No. 4 Ferr Phos | for chills, fevers, inflammation, congestion, coughs and colds | iron phosphate |
| – No. 5 Kali Mur | respiratory ailments, coughs, colds and children's feverish complaints | potassium chloride |
| – No. 9 Nat Mur | for watery colds, flow of tears and loss of taste and smell | sodium chloride |
| – No. 11 Nat. Sulph | influenza | sodium sulphate |
| – Combination J | coughs, colds and chestiness | iron phosphate, potassium chloride, sodium chloride |

| Products | Uses | Ingredients |
|---|---|---|

– Combination Q  catarrh and sinus disorders

iron phosphate, potassium chloride, potassium sulphate, sodium chloride

## Anthroposophical

Wala Pillules
– Archangelica Comp.　laryngitis, hoarseness, tickly coughs　angelica

– Berberis/Quartz　symptomatic relief of blocked sinuses　barberry, silicon dioxide

– Gelsemium Comp.　symptomatic relief of flu' and head colds　gelsemium

– Silicea Comp.　symptomatic relief of head colds　silicon dioxide

Weleda
– Aconitum/Bryonia Drops　for relief of colds and flu'　aconite, white bryony

– Bolus Eucalypti Comp. Gargle Powder　for relief of sore throats and tonsillitis　apis mel, belladonna, eucalyptus, kaolin

– Cough Elixir　a natural expectorant　aniseed, horehound, thyme, marshmallow, sundew, ipecac. pasque flower, malt extract

– Catarrh Cream　to relieve nasal congestion　horse chestnut, berberis, blackthorn, white bryony, camphor, echinacea, eucalyptus, peppermint, thyme

– Cinnabar 20x Tablets　for catarrh and recurrent sore throats　cinnabar

– Cinnabar 20x/Pyrites 3x　for sore throats　cinnabar, pyrites

– Cough Drops　for dry and irritating coughs　angelica, cinnamon, clove, coriander, lemon, lemon balm, nutmeg, cherry laurel

– Erysidoron 1　for sore throats　apis mel, belladonna

– Erysidoron 2　for sore throats　charcoal, sulphur

– Oleum Rhinale Nasal Drops　for catarrh and sinus congestion　marigold, peppermint, eucalyptus, mercurius sulphuratus ruber

– Pyrites 3x Tablets　for sore throat, hoarseness, loss of voice　pyrites

| Products | Uses | Ingredients |
|---|---|---|

## Allopathic

| Products | Uses | Ingredients |
|---|---|---|
| Codeine Linctus BP | for relief of dry coughs | codeine |
| Eucalyptus Oil BP | for relief of catarrh, muscular sprains, cramps | eucalyptus |
| Gee's Linctus BP | for relief of coughs | opium, squill, benzoic acid |
| Glycerin BP | for sore throats, rough and chapped skin | glycerin |
| Glycerin, Lemon and Honey | for relief of cough and sore throat | glycerol, lemon, honey, citric acid |
| Ipecacuanha and Morphine Mixture BP 1980 | for relief of stubborn coughs | morphine, ipecacuanha, liquorice, treacle, peppermint |
| Menthol and Eucalyptus Inhalation BP | an inhalation for colds and catarrh | menthol, eucalyptus, magnesium carbonate |
| Simple Linctus BP | for relief of coughs | citric acid |
| Allen's – Chesty Cough | for chesty coughs | ammonium chloride, tolu, squill, menthol, horehound |
| – Dry Cough | for dry tickly coughs | benzoin, ipecacuanha, capsicum |
| – Pine and Honey Balsam | for coughs, cold and bronchitis | ipecacuanha, liquorice, pumilio pine, squill |
| – Junior Cough Syrup | for tickly coughs and sore throats | glycerin, citric acid |
| Beehive Balsam | for stubborn coughs | honey, glycerin, ipecacuanha, lemon |
| Bronalin Decongestant | for blocked sinuses, stuffed up noses and catarrh | pseudoephedrine |
| Buttercup Syrup – Original | for coughs, colds, sore throats | squill, capsicum |
| – Honey and Lemon | for chesty, bronchial, dry or tickly coughs | ipecacuanha, glucose, menthol, honey |
| – Infant Cough Syrup | for relief of children's coughs | ipecacuanha, glucose, menthol |

| Products | Uses | Ingredients |
|---|---|---|
| Cam | for treatment of broncho-spasm, bronchitis | ephedrine |
| Contac Non-drowsy | decongestant for colds, flu' and allergy | pseudoephedrine |
| Covonia Mentholated | for relief of productive coughs | menthol, squill, liquorice |
| Do-Do Chesteze Tablets | for relief of bronchial cough, wheezing and breathlessness and clear chest of mucus | ephedrine, theophylline |
| Famel Original | for dry, troublesome coughs | creosote, codeine |
| Fennings Little Healers | aid to expectoration in coughs | ipecacuanha, lactose |
| Galloway's Cough Syrup | for coughs and hoarseness | ipecacuanha, squill |
| Galpseud Linctus and Tablets | for relief of nasal, sinus and upper respiratory congestion | pseudoephedrine |
| Hacks | for relief of coughs and colds | menthol, eucalyptus |
| Hall's | | |
| – Mentholyptus | for sore throat, colds, congestion | menthol, eucalytpus |
| – Soothers | for sore throat, colds, congestion | menthol, eucalyptus |
| Happinose | for relief of nasal congestion in colds, catarrh, head colds and hay fever | menthol, essential oils |
| Hill's Balsam | | |
| – Chesty Cough/Children | for chesty cough and catarrh | ipecacuanha, citric acid |
| – Chesty Cough Pastilles | for chesty coughs, colds, catarrh | benzoin, peppermint, ipecacuanha, menthol |
| – Extra Strong 2in1 Pastilles | for coughs, colds, catarrh | benzoin, ipecacuanha, menthol, peppermint |
| – Nasal Congestion Pastilles | for relief of nasal congestion | menthol, eucalyptus |

# C

| Products | Uses | Ingredients |
|---|---|---|
| J. Collis Browne's Mixture | for alleviation of coughs | morphine, peppermint |
| Jackson's<br>– Lemon Linctus | for relief of coughs and sore throat | honey, glycerol |
| – Mentholated Balm | relieves nasal congestion, muscular pains and stiffness | eucalyptus, methyl salicylate, camphor, terpineol, menthol |
| – Troublesome Cough | for coughs | honey, glycerol, ipecacuanha |
| Karvol | for relief of nasal congestion and head colds | levomenthol, chlorbutol, pine oils, terpineol, thymol |
| Karvol Vapour Rub | helps clear nasal congestion | pine, eucalyptus, menthol |
| Kilkof | for coughs, colds, sore throat | benzoin, ipecacuanha, capsicum |
| Lemsip Dry Cough | for dry coughs and sore throats | lemon, glycerol, citric acid, syrup |
| Lockets<br>– Lozenges | for relief of blocked nose and sore throat | menthol, eucalyptus, honey, glycerol |
| – Medicated Linctus | for relief of coughs and sore throats | glycerol, honey, glucose, ipecacuanha |
| Meggazones Pastilles | for sore throats, coughs, colds, catarrh | menthol |
| Meltus Baby Cough Linctus | for coughs associated with colds | acetic acid |
| Mentholatum<br>– Antiseptic Lozenges | for coughs, head colds, congestion | menthol, eucalyptus |
| – Vapour Rub | for colds, catarrh, hay fever, muscular aches and pains | menthol, camphor, methyl salicylate |
| Nostroline | for soothing relief of blocked noses | menthol, eucalyptus, geranium |

| Products | Uses | Ingredients |
|----------|------|-------------|
| Olbas | | |
| – Oil | for bronchial and nasal congestion due to colds, catarrh, flu', hay fever, rhinitis | cajuput, clove, eucalyptus, juniper, menthol, wintergreen |
| – Pastilles | for coughs, colds, catarrh, sore throat, influenza and headache due to congestion | eucalyptus, peppermint, clove, menthol, juniper, wintergreen |
| – Inhaler | for relief of blocked sinuses, colds, catarrh, hay fever and influenza | cajuput, eucalyptus, levomethol, peppermint |
| Potter's | | |
| – Catarrh Pastilles | for colds, coughs and catarrh | pumilio pine, eucalyptus, creosote, menthol |
| – Decongestant Pastilles | for blocked noses, coughs, catarrh | menthol, eucalyptus |
| – Gee's Linctus Pastilles | for coughs | opium, squill, cinnamic acid, benzoic acid, acetic acid, honey |
| – Strong Bronchial Catarrh Pastilles | for bronchial catarrh, coughs, colds | menthol, benzoin, aniseed, peppermint, capsaicin creosote |
| – Sugar-Free Cough Pastilles | for coughs, colds and catarrh | liquorice, menthol, benzoin, aniseed, clove, peppermint, capsicum |
| Pulmo Bailly | for coughs with catarrh | guaiacol, codeine |
| Secron Syrup | for nasal congestion with children's colds, catarrh, chesty coughs | ephedrine, ipecacuanha |
| Snufflebabe | for congestion in babies | eucalyptus, thyme |
| Sudafed Elixir and Tablets | for cold and flu' symptoms, hay fever | pseudoephedrine |
| Throaties | for coughs and colds | benzoin, menthol |
| Tixylix | | |
| – Baby Syrup | for relief of dry tickly coughs | glycerol |
| – Colds and Hayfever Inhalant Capsules | for relief of blocked nose and congestion with colds, catarrh, flu', hay fever | menthol, eucalyptus, camphor, turpentine |

| Products | Uses | Ingredients |
|---|---|---|
| Veno's | | |
| – Dry Cough | for dry coughs | glucose, treacle |
| – Honey and Lemon | for tickly coughs | lemon, honey, glucose |
| Vick's | | |
| – Nasal Stick | for relief of nasal congestion | menthol, camphor, pine |
| – Vaporub | for relief of nasal catarrh and congestion due to colds, sore throat and cough | menthol, camphor, eucalyptus, turpentine |
| – Vaposyrup/ Tickly Cough | for relief of dry, tickly coughs | menthol |
| Woodward's Baby Chest Rub | for relief of catarrh and congestion due to colds | turpentine, eucalyptus, menthol |
| Vocalzones | for irritation due to speaking or smoking | menthol, peppermint, myrrh |
| Zubes | | |
| – Original | for coughs, colds and sore throats | menthol, aniseed, |
| – Honey and Lemon | for coughs, colds and sore throats | honey, lemon, citric acid, menthol |
| – Blackcurrant | for children's coughs | citric acid, menthol, aniseed |

# Constipation

Constipation is the infrequent passage of hard, dry stools. Bowel habits vary from one person to another – regular may mean twice a day or twice a week.

Stimulant laxatives, such as senna, increase the speed at which the contents move through the bowel. Osmotic laxatives, such as magnesium sulphate, act by drawing extra fluid into the bowel, producing softer stools. Bulk laxatives, such as bran, ispaghula and sterculia, take longer to work but are useful for those with haemorrhoids and for some with irritable bowel syndrome, as they soften the stools and make them easier to pass. An increased fluid intake will also help those who suffer from constipation.

Some products are either not recommended, or have a reduced dosage, in pregnancy or whilst breast-feeding. There are also reduced doses for children, although they should be seen by the doctor if the problem persists.

| Products | Uses | Ingredients |
| --- | --- | --- |
| **Herbal** | | |
| Califig Herbal Tablets | for relief of constipation | dandelion, peppermint, senna |
| Calsalettes | for relief of constipation | aloin |
| Dorwest Natural Herb Tablets | for occasional constipation | senna, aloe, cascara, valerian, dandelion |
| Fam-Lax Senna Tablets | for relief of occasional constipation | rhubarb, senna, irish moss |
| Gerard House Herbulax | for relief of occasional constipation | buckthorn, dandelion |
| Heath and Heather Inner Fresh Laxative Tablets | for occasional constipation | buckthorn |
| Herbal Concepts Laxative Tablets | for short-term relief of constipation | aloes, cascara, senna, valerian |
| Jackson's Herbal Laxative | for relief of occasional constipation | cascara, rhubarb, senna |
| Lane's Dual-Lax Tablets | for temporary constipation | senna, alion, cascara |

| Products | Uses | Ingredients |
|---|---|---|
| Lusty's Herbalene Herbal | for temporary or occasional constipation | senna, buckthorn, elder, fennel |
| Modern Herbals Laxative Tablets | for temporary constipation | senna, aloin, cascara |
| Potter's | | |
| – Lion Cleansing Herbs | for occasional constipation | buckthorn, ispaghula, senna, elder, fennel, maté |
| – Lion Cleansing Tablets | for occasional constipation | senna, aloes, cascara, dandelion, fennel |
| – Out of Sorts | for occasional constipation | senna, aloes, cascara, dandelion, fennel |
| Sure-Lax (Herbal) | for occasional or non-persistent constipation | valerian, holy thistle, fennel, aloes |
| Weleda Clairo Tea | for occasional or non-persistent constipation | aniseed, clove, peppermint, senna |

## Homoeopathic

| bryonia | for stools that feel too large to pass | bryony |
|---|---|---|
| graphites | for constipation with colicky pains | graphite |
| lycopodium | for constipation with flatulence, hard stools | club moss |
| nux vom | for constipation with frequent urge but feel more to come | nux vomica |
| sulphur | for painful, large, hard, dry stools | sulphur |

## Anthroposophical

| Weleda Laxadoron Tablets | gentle laxative | caraway, clove, century, yarrow, peppermint, senna, aniseed, wax plant nectar |
|---|---|---|

## Allopathic

| Castor Oil BP | for relief of occasional constipation | castor oil |
|---|---|---|
| Liquid Paraffin BP | for relief of occasional constipation | liquid paraffin |

| Products | Uses | Ingredients |
|----------|------|-------------|
| Califig | for relief of constipation | senna, fig |
| Califig Junior | to promote bowel regularity | fig |
| Ex-Lax Senna | for temporary relief of constipation | senna |
| Fybogel | for constipation, restoration of regularity | ispaghula |
| Fynnon Salts | for relief of constipation | sodium sulphate |
| Isogel | for constipation, diarrhoea, irritable bowel | ispaghula |
| Juno Junipah Salts | for temporary relief of constipation | sodium sulphate, phosphate and bicarbonate, juniper |
| Kest | for temporary relief of constipation | magnesium sulphate |
| Konsyl | for constipation, irritable bowel, diarrhoea | ispaghula |
| Manevac | for constipation, bowel regulation | ispaghula, senna |
| Normacol | for constipation | sterculia |
| Normacol Plus | for constipation | sterculia, buckthorn |
| Nylax with Senna | for relief of occasional constipation | senna |
| Potter's Senna Tablets | for relief and prevention of constipation | senna |
| Regulan | for constipation and increase fibre intake | ispaghula |
| Senokot | for relief of occasional constipation | senna |
| Sure-Lax Senna | for constipation | senna |

# Diarrhoea

Diarrhoea is usually caused by viruses or bacteria, ingested with contaminated food or drink. It can also be caused by change of climate, stress, hot spicy food, too much alcohol, and by certain medicines, such as antibiotics.

It should be treated by fasting (eating no food) for 24 hours but drinking plenty of water and soft (non-fizzy) drinks. Milk should also be avoided as it can cause further upset.

It is most important, especially with the very young and very old, that dehydration does not occur; oral rehydration products in various flavours are available from your local pharmacy.

Adsorbents, such as kaolin and attapulgite, work by adsorbing the toxins produced by bacteria. Opiates like morphine and codeine delay intestinal transit time so allowing more water to be absorbed from the stools. Belladonna is antispasmodic and reduces the activity of the colon.

| Products | Uses | Ingredients |
|---|---|---|
| **Herbal** | | |
| Potter's Spanish Tummy Mixture | for non-persistent diarrhoea | blackberry, catechu |
| Weleda Melissa Comp. | for nausea, stomach ache, stomach upsets and occasional diarrhoea | lemon balm, nutmeg, cinnamon, angelica, lemon oil, coriander, clove |
| **Homoeopathic** | | |
| aconite | for sudden onset diarrhoea after shock or cold wind | aconite |
| argent nit | for diarrhoea due to excitement or apprehension | silver nitrate |
| arsen alb | for diarrhoea from food poisoning, holiday diarrhoea | arsenic trioxide |
| colocynthis | for diarrhoea with spasmodic griping pains | bitter cucumber |
| pulsatilla | for diarrhoea, worse at night, from cold drinks and fatty foods | pasque flower |

| Products | Uses | Ingredients |
|---|---|---|
| sulphur | for diarrhoea with urge to open bowels early in morning | sulphur |

## Allopathic

| | | |
|---|---|---|
| Kaolin Mixture BP | for relief of diarrhoea | kaolin, sodium bicarbonate |
| Kaolin Paediatric Mixture BP | for relief of diarrhoea in children | kaolin |
| Kaolin and Morphine Mixture BP | for relief of diarrhoea and upset stomachs | kaolin, sodium bicarbonate, morphine |
| Diocalm Dual Action | for occasional diarrhoea and associated pain and discomfort | morphine, attapulgite |
| Dioralyte | to replace fluid and electrolyte loss in vomiting and diarrhoea | sodium and potassium salts, glucose |
| Electrolade | oral rehydration therapy for electrolyte and fluid loss due to diarrhoea | sodium and potassium salts, glucose |
| Entrocalm Tablets | for diarrhoea and holiday tummy | kaolin |
| Entrocalm Replace | electrolye replacement therapy | sodium and potassium salts, dextrose |
| J. Collis Browne's Mixture | for alleviation of diarrhoea | morphine, peppermint |
| – Tablets | for relief of occasional diarrhoea | kaolin, morphine, calcium carbonate |
| Kao – C | for diarrhoea | kaolin, calcium carbonate, carminative oils |
| Kaodene | for acute diarrhoea | codeine, kaolin |
| Opazimes | for upset stomach, diarrhoea, mild gastroenteritis | aluminium hydroxide, kaolin, belladonna, morphine |
| Rehidrat | for diarrhoea and associated dehydration | sodium and potassium salts, citric acid, sugars |

# Ears

Ears are precious. Never poke anything into the ear, because it may impact the wax or puncture the ear drum.

To soften earwax is the only ear treatment that does not need to be dealt with by a doctor. Any pain, swelling or deafness in the ear needs to be checked out by a doctor.

| Products | Uses | Ingredients |
| --- | --- | --- |

### Homoeopathic

| Products | Uses | Ingredients |
| --- | --- | --- |
| aconite | for earache after exposure to cold, dry winds | aconite |
| belladonna | for throbbing earache made worse by warmth | belladonna |
| chamomilla | for painful, irritable, weepy earache | chamomile |
| hepar sulph | for throbbing earache, better with warmth | calcium sulphide |
| pulsatilla | for swollen red ear, patient weepy | pasque flower |

### Allopathic

| Products | Uses | Ingredients |
| --- | --- | --- |
| Sodium Bicarbonate Ear Drops BP | to soften earwax | sodium bicarbonate |
| Ear Calm Spray | for superficial infection of outer ear | acetic acid |
| Earex | for earwax softening and removal | arachis, almond, camphor |
| Soothol Earache Drops | for softening earwax | cajuput, rosemary, arachis |
| Waxwane | softens hard wax before syringing | turpentine, terpineol |

# Eyes

Eyes are very precious and should be treated with great care. Any eye condition that does not improve, or is getting worse after two or three days should be seen by a doctor urgently.

Any sudden pain or blurring of vision should also be treated urgently.

Eye lotions are soothing preparations which are useful for minor irritation caused by a dusty or smoky atmosphere, driving or overwork. Preparations for dry eyes are useful for the elderly, in whom dry eye is common, as it is often associated with connective tissue diseases, like arthritis.

Contact lens wearers should check pack information carefully as many products will not be suitable for them, particularly those wearing soft lenses.

Eye preparations should be discarded four weeks after first opening.

| Products | Uses | Ingredients |
|---|---|---|
| **Homoeopathic** | | |
| apis mel | for recurring styes, red, swollen painful eyelids | honey-bee |
| arnica | for tired eyes | arnica |
| hepar sulph | for styes with pus | calcium sulphide |
| nat mur | for eye ache looking up, down or to sides | sodium chloride |
| phosphorus | for tired eyes from nervous apprehension | phosphoric acid |
| pulsatilla | for conjuctivitis | pasque flower |
| ruta grav | for tired eyes, burning after close work or study | rue |
| thuja | for dry, scaly eyelids stuck together overnight | white cedar |

E

| Products | Uses | Ingredients |
|---|---|---|

## Anthroposophical

Weleda Larch Resin
| – Compound Lotion | for tired eyes | pineapple, lavender, larch, acacia |
| – Ointment | for tired eyes | pineapple, lavender, larch |

## Allopathic

| Simple Eye Ointment BP | to lubricate and protect the eyes | yellow soft and liquid paraffin lanolin |
| Lacrilube | to lubricate and protect the eyes | white soft and liquid paraffin, lanolin alcohols |
| Lubri-Tears | to lubricate and protect the eyes | white soft and liquid paraffin, lanolin |

Optrex
| – Eye Drops | for relief of minor eye irritation | witch hazel |
| – Lotion | for relief of minor eye irritation | witch hazel |

# Feet – Athelete's Foot, Corns, Calluses, Warts and Verrucas

Athlete's foot is an unsightly, irritating and smelly foot condition which is caused by a fungal infection. The fungus, Tinea pedis, likes to live in warm, moist places, like feet.

It is contagious and can be picked up by simply walking over a damp floor, as in communal showers or swimming baths. Treatment with antifungal cream or ointment should continue for at least a week or two after the infection seems to have cleared up to ensure that it has really been cured. An antifungal powder should be sprinkled into every pair of shoes to kill the spores produced by the fungus and so prevent re-infection at a later date.

Corns and calluses are areas of hard, thickened skin, which are caused by badly fitting footwear and will recur if the cause is not attended to.

Warts and verrucas are caused by a viral infection. Verrucas are also called plantar warts as they are simply warts on the sole of the foot. Warts can occur anywhere on the body. They are contagious and are commonly picked up at schools, sports centres and swimming baths. The treatments, which are not suitable for use on the face or genital area, contain skin-dissolving ingredients. Treatment of warts and verrucas can take some time, with daily application of the medication after removal of the previous day's dead tissue with a pumice stone.

Diabetics and others with circulatory disorders should never treat their corns, calluses, warts or verrucas: they should see the chiropodist at their local hospital for treatment.

Caution should be exercised by those sensitive to salicylates, including aspirin, such as asthmatics, as most of these products contain salicylates.

| Products | Uses | Ingredients |
|---|---|---|
| **Herbal** | | |
| Lane's Balto Foot Balm | for tired, aching feet, softens hard cracked skin | camphor, menthol, zinc oxide, sulphur |
| Modern Herbals Foot Balm | for tired, aching feet, softens hard cracked skin | camphor, menthol, zinc oxide, sulphur |

# F

| Products | Uses | Ingredients |
|---|---|---|

## Allopathic

| Products | Uses | Ingredients |
|---|---|---|
| Compound Benzoic Acid (Whitfield's) Ointment BP | for treatment of athlete's foot, ringworm | benzoic acid, salicylic acid |
| Bazuka | for corns, calluses, verrucas, warts | salicylic acid, lactic acid |
| Carnation | | |
| – Corn Caps | for treatment of corns | salicylic acid |
| – Callous Caps | for treatment of calluses | salicylic acid |
| – Verruca Care | for treatment of verrucas | salicylic acid |
| Compound W | for treatment of warts and verrucas | salicylic acid |
| Cuplex Gel | for corns, calluses, warts | salicylic acid, lactic acid |
| Duofilm | for warts and verrucas | salicylic acid, lactic acid |
| Occlusal | for warts and verrucas | salicylic acid |
| Pickles | | |
| – Corn Caps | for treatment of corns | salicylic acid, colophony |
| – Foot Ointment | for corns and hard skin | salicylic acid |
| Salatac – Gel | for warts, corns and calluses | salicylic acid, camphor, lactic acid, pyroxylin |
| Salactol Wart Paint | for warts and verrucas | salicylic acid, lactic acid |
| Scholl | | |
| – Corn and Callus Removal Liquid | to remove corns and calluses | salicylic acid, camphor |
| – Corn Removal Plasters | to remove corns | salicylic acid |
| – Callus Removal Pads | to remove callusses | salicylic acid |
| – Heal and Seal Verruca Gel | for warts and verrucas | salicylic acid, camphor |
| – Verruca Removal System | for warts and verrucas | salicylic acid |
| Toepedo Cream | for treatment of athlete's foot | salicylic acid, benzoic acid |
| Verrugon Complete | for verrucas | salicylic acid |
| Wartex Ointment | for hard and ragged warts | salicylic acid |

# First Aid

Cuts and grazes are best treated by washing the wound before applying an antiseptic cream and a plaster. Burns and scalds should be held under running cold water for at least ten minutes. Severe burns involving broken skin need medical attention, as does any burn on a child, and for adults too if it is larger than the palm of the hand. Mild sunburn can be treated with cooling baths and application of cooling creams, lotions and ointments. With sunburn, plenty of water should be drunk to avoid dehydration; also avoid alcohol as this may cause further dehydration. Severe sunburn, which causes dehydration, fever and vomiting needs medical attention.

Insect bites and stings can be treated with creams or sprays. Bees leave their sting behind when they sting – this should be removed, taking care not to squeeze the poison sack attached to the sting. Anyone who suffers wheezing or breathlessness after a wasp or bee sting should seek medical attention immediately, for this allergic response. Those who already know they are allergic should always carry an Epipen with which they can inject adrenaline before seeking further medical advice.

| Products | Uses | Ingredients |
|---|---|---|
| **Herbal** | | |
| Potter's – Comfrey Ointment | for bruises and strains | comfrey, lanolin |
| Dermacreme Ointment | a mild antiseptic for cuts, grazes, minor burns and scalds | menthol, methyl salicylate, phenol, starch, zinc oxide, yellow soft paraffin, lanolin |
| Savlon Natural First Aid – for Burns | treatment for minor burns and scalds | nettle, marigold, echinacea, st john's wort |
| – for Cuts and Sores | treatment of cuts and sores | st john's wort, marigold |
| – for Insect Bites and Stings | treatment for insect bites and stings | st john's wort, yellow dock, echinacea, marsh tea, marigold, arnica, pyrethrum |

| Products | Uses | Ingredients |
|---|---|---|
| Weleda | | |
| – Arnica Ointment | for muscular pain, stiffness, sprains, bruises and swellings after contusions | arnica, lanolin, beeswax, wool alcohols, olive and sunflower oils |
| – Arnica Lotion | for muscular pain, stiffness, sprains, bruises | arnica |
| – Calendula Lotion | for cuts, minor wounds and abrasions | marigold |
| – Hypericum/Calendula Ointment | for symptomatic relief of painful cuts and minor wounds | marigold, st john's wort, lanolin, wool alcohols, olive and sunflower oils, beeswax |

## Homoeopathic

| | | |
|---|---|---|
| aconite | for shock, fear and panic after an accident | aconite |
| apis mel | for insect stings | honey-bee |
| arnica | for all injuries that lead to bruising | arnica |
| belladonna | for sunburn with redness, heat and throbbing | belladonna |
| cantharis | to aid healing of burns and scalds | spanish fly |
| hepar sulph | for puncture wounds showing signs of infection | calcium sulphide |
| hypericum | for painful crush injuries, horsefly bites | st john's wort |
| ledum | for pain from puncture wounds of small sharp objects | marsh tea |
| ruta grav | for sprains where the bone is bruised | rue |
| symphytum | for injuries to bones and tendons | comfrey |
| urtica urens | for stinging burns and scalds | nettle |
| Nelson's | | |
| – Arnica Cream | for bruises | arnica |
| – Burns Ointment | for burns and scalds – for relief of pain blistering and speedy healing | marigold, nettle, echinacea, st johns wort |
| – Hypercal Spray | for cuts and sores | st john's wort, marigold |

| Products | Uses | Ingredients |
|---|---|---|
| – Pyrethrum Spray | for insect bites and stings | st john's wort, echinacea, marsh tea, marigold, arnica, yellow dock, pyrethrum |
| – Tea Tree Cream | antiseptic | tea tree |

## Anthroposophical

Weleda

| | | |
|---|---|---|
| – Arnica 6x Tablets | for shock and accidental upset | arnica |
| – Combudoron Lotion | for minor burns | arnica, nettle |
| – Ointment | for minor burns and scalds | arnica, nettle |
| – Spray | for insect bites | arnica, nettle |
| – Calendolon Ointment | for treatment of cuts, minor wounds and abrasions | marigold |

## Allopathic

| | | |
|---|---|---|
| Calamine Lotion BP | for rashes and sunburn | calamine, zinc oxide, bentonite |
| Compound Calamine and Cream BPC | for relief of itching and skin irritation and mild sunburn | calamine, zinc oxide, liquid yellow soft paraffin, lanolin |
| Oily Calamine Lotion BP | for mild sunburn and other skin conditions | calamine, calcium hydroxide, lanolin, oleic acid, arachis oil |
| Iodine Tincture BP | for use as an antiseptic | iodine, potassium iodide, alcohol |
| Betadine Antiseptic Paint | for cuts, grazes, abrasions | iodine |
| – Cream, Ointment and Spray | for cuts, grazes and minor burns | iodine |
| Germolene Antiseptic Ointment | for minor cuts, grazes, burns, scalds | lanolin, yellow and white soft and liquid paraffin, starch, zinc oxide, methyl salicylate, phenol |

| Products | Uses | Ingredients |
|---|---|---|
| Lacto Calamine Lotion | for sunburn, insect bites, stings | calamine, zinc oxide, witch hazel, phenol |
| Witch Skin Treatment Gel | for minor rashes, irritation, sunburn | witch hazel |

# Haemorrhoids

Haemorrhoids, commonly called piles, are varicose veins that occur in or around the rectum and anus. They cause irritation, itching and pain, and the preparations listed will help. Good toilet hygiene is also important. Moist toilet tissues are available. Bleeding piles should be seen by a doctor. Constipation is a major cause of haemorrhoids: increasing the amount of fibre in the diet will help to soften the stools and make them easier to pass.

| Products | Uses | Ingredients |
|---|---|---|
| **Herbal** | | |
| Lane's | | |
| – Heemex Pile Ointment | relief of discomfort, itching and irritation | witch hazel, benzoin, zinc oxide |
| – Pileabs Tablets | for temporary constipation and itching, irritation and discomfort of piles | slippery elm, cascara |
| Modern Herbals | | |
| – Pile Ointment | relief of discomfort, itching and irritation due to piles | witch hazel, benzoin, zinc oxide |
| – Pile Tablets | for temporary constipation and itching, irritation and discomfort of piles | slippery elm, cascara |
| Potter's | | |
| – Green Pilewort Ointment | piles | pilewort |
| – Piletabs | haemorrhoids aggravated by constipation | pilewort, agrimony, cascara, stoneroot |

| Products | Uses | Ingredients |
|---|---|---|

## Homoeopathic

| | | |
|---|---|---|
| calc fluor | for symptomatic relief of haemorrhoids | calcium fluoride |
| graphites | for anal fissure, sore, smarting pain when passing stools | graphite |
| hamamelis | for bleeding piles, anus sore and bruised | witch hazel |
| nux vom | for large piles that burn and sting | nux vomica |
| pulsatilla | for painful piles that bleed easily | pasque flower |
| sulphur | for piles that do not bleed but are aggravated by warmth | sulphur |
| Nelson's Haemorrhoid Cream | haemorrhoids | horse chestnut, marigold, witch hazel, peony |
| New Era Tissue Salts: | | |
| – No.1 Calc Fluor | for maintaining tissue elasticity and for impaired circulation, varicose veins and piles | calcium fluoride |
| – Combination G | for piles | calcium fluoride, calcium phosphate, potassium phosphate, sodium chloride |

## Anthroposophical

| | | |
|---|---|---|
| Weleda Antimony Ointment | for relief of external haemorrhoids | antimony |

## Allopathic

| | | |
|---|---|---|
| Preparation H – Ointment | for relief of pain, irritation and itching | yeast cell extract, shark-liver oil |
| – Suppositories | for relief of pain, irritation and itching | yeast cell extract, shark-liver oil |
| – Clear Gel | for relief of pain irritation and itching | witch hazel |

# Hair and Scalp

Dandruff is the most common scalp condition, and severe cases may be referred to as seborrhoeic dermatitis. Eczema and psoriasis may also occur on the scalp.

Cradle cap is a type of dermatitis where the baby's scalp is scaly with crusting; this occurs in the first few months of life and usually resolves itself before the baby's first birthday.

| Products | Uses | Ingredients |
| --- | --- | --- |
| **Herbal** | | |
| Potter's | | |
| – Adiantine | improves hair, eliminates dandruff | bay, rosemary, witch hazel |
| – Medicated Extract of Rosemary | to improve hair condition | rosegeranium, rosemary, bay, methyl salicylate |
| **Homoeopathic** | | |
| nat mur | for greasy hair, flaking skin at hairline | sodium chloride |
| sulphur | dry, flaking scalp, with burning and itching | sulphur |
| New Era Tissue Salts: | | |
| – No. 7 Kali Sulph | for falling hair | potassium sulphate |
| – No. 12 Silica | for lacklustre hair | silicon dioxide |
| – Combination K | for brittle nails and falling hair | potassium sulphate, sodium chloride, silicon dioxide |
| **Allopathic** | | |
| Alphosyl 2 in 1 | for scalp psoriasis, seborrhoeic dermatitis dandruff and itching scalp | coal tar |
| Betadine Shampoo | for seborrheic conditions, infected scalp | iodine |

| | | |
|---|---|---|
| Capasal Shampoo | for dry, scaly scalp conditions including seborrhoeic dermatitis, psoriasis, cradle cap | salicylic acid, coconut, coal tar |
| Clinitar Shampoo | for scalp psoriasis, seborrhoeic dermatitis and dandruff | coal tar |
| Cocois Coconut Oil Compound | treatment of scaly scalp conditions, eczema, psoriasis, seborrhoeic dermatitis, dandruff | coal tar, sulphur, salicylic acid, coconut |
| Gelcotar Liquid | for scalp psoriasis, seborrhoeic dermatitis, dandruff | coal tar, cade oil |
| Meted Shampoo | for seborrhoeic dermatitis, scalp psoriasis, severe dandruff | salicylic acid, sulphur |
| Pentrax Shampoo | for seborrhoeic dermatitis, scalp psoriasis, severe dandruff | coal tar |
| Polytar Liquid | for scalp disorders such as psoriasis, dandruff, seborrhoea, eczema, itching | pine, cade, coal tar, arachis, oleyl alcohol |
| Pragmatar Cream | for cradle cap, seborrhoeic conditions | coal tar, salicylic acid |
| Psoriderm Scalp Lotion | for psoriasis of the scalp | coal tar, lecithin |
| T/Gel Shampoo | treats itchy, flaky scalp disorders such as psoriasis, dandruff, seborrhoeic dermatitis | coal tar |
| SCR | for cradle cap | salicylic acid |

# Hay Fever

About 12 million people in the United Kingdom suffer from hay fever, and this number is thought to be increasing. Hay fever is caused by the body's allergic response to pollen from trees, grasses and other plants, and the spores produced by moulds and fungi. Hay fever causes a variety of symptoms: sneezing, watering eyes, runny nose and nasal congestion, itching of the nose and sometimes of the roof of the mouth, headache and tiredness. The symptoms may only occur at a particular time of year, depending on which pollen is causing the allergy.

Some of the products listed should not be taken in pregnancy or while breast-feeding.

| Products | Uses | Ingredients |
|---|---|---|
| **Herbal** | | |
| Herbal Concepts Hay Fever and Sinus Relief | hay fever, catarrh and sinus congestion | echinacea, elder flower, garlic |
| HRI Garlic Tablets | catarrh and rhinitis | garlic |
| Lane's Herbelix Specific | catarrh, hay fever, rhinitis, mucous congestion and head cold | lobelia, tolu and sodium bicarbonate |
| Modern Herbals Cold and Congestion Syrup | catarrh, hay fever, rhinitis, mucous congestion and head cold | lobelia, tolu and sodium bicarbonate |
| Lusty's Garlic Perles | catarrh, rhinitis, common cold | garlic |

**Homoeopathic**

| | | |
|---|---|---|
| allium cepa | for streaming eyes and nose, sneezing, worse in morning indoors | onion |
| arsen alb | for violent, painful sneezing and watery discharge making upper lip sore | arsenic trioxide |
| euphrasia | for itchy, sore, burning eyes and runny nose | eyebright |
| gelsemium | for non-stop sneezing, puffy watery eyes | gelsemium |
| mixed pollen | a general remedy for allergic response to pollen | |

| Products | Uses | Ingredients |
|---|---|---|
| nat mur | for copious catarrh and sneezing with cold sores | sodium chloride |
| nux vom | for sneezing and irritation of nose, eyes, throat | nux vomica |
| pulsatilla | for thick catarrh and sneezing, relieved by open air | pasque flower |
| silicea | for sinusitis, blocked, stuffy nose, worse on waking | silicon dioxide |
| Nelson's Pollenna | hay fever | onion, eyebright, sabadilla |
| New Era Tissue Salts – Combination H | hay fever, allergic rhinitis | magnesium phosphate, sodium chloride, silicon dioxide |

## Anthroposophical

| | | |
|---|---|---|
| Weleda Gencydo Ointment | for hay fever symptoms | quince, lemon |

# Indigestion, Flatulence, Heartburn, Colic, Irritable Bowel

Indigestion is a term used to describe a number of conditions. The most common symptoms are pain, nausea, flatulence, bloating and even vomiting. It may be caused by eating too much, or by rich, spicy food, incomplete digestion of food, or delayed emptying of the food from the stomach. Greasy foods, coffee, chocolate and alcohol should be avoided by those prone to indigestion. Some medicines may irritate the stomach lining, for example aspirin, ibuprofen.

Irritable bowel syndrome is three times as common in women than in men. It can be caused by stress, change of diet or an infection. The symptoms include abdominal pain, bloating, diarrhoea, constipation, excessive wind and rectal discomfort. Treatments include peppermint oil, which is carminative and antispasmodic, and hyoscine which relaxes smooth muscle of the bowel. Some fibre products, also used as laxatives, are used to treat irritable bowel syndrome.

Some antacids should not be taken at the same time of day as some antibiotics – read the label on antibiotics carefully – it will tell you if this is the case.

Some of the products listed should be avoided by those with kidney problems. And those with high blood pressure or heart problems should not take products with a high sodium content. Those with glaucoma should also check with their pharmacist.

Many of these products are suitable for use in pregnancy but a few are not. The advice of a pharmacist should be sought as to the most appropriate remedy.

| Products | Uses | Ingredients |
| --- | --- | --- |
| **Herbal** | | |
| Bio-Strath Artichoke Formula | for relief of indigestion after eating fatty food | artichoke, thistle, peppermint, yeast |
| Dorwest Digestive Tablets | for indigestion, heartburn, hyperacidity and nausea | ginger, golden seal, rhubarb, valerian |
| Gerard House Slippery Elm Tablets | aids digestion and relieves the symptoms of gastric disorders | slippery elm |

| Products | Uses | Ingredients |
|---|---|---|
| Herbal Concepts<br>– Indigestion Relief | for relief of indigestion, nausea and colic associated with fatty meals | black root, capsicum, fringe tree, ginger |
| – Wind and Dyspepsia Relief | for relief of flatulence and nervous dyspepsia | ginger, goldenseal, myrrh, rhubarb, valerian, dandelion |
| HRI Golden Seal Digestive Tablets | to aid digestion and relieve flatulence | ginger, myrrh, golden-seal, rhubarb, valerian |
| Lane's Charcoal Tablets | for flatulence, indigestion and heartburn including dyspepsia and occasional diarrhoea | charcoal |
| Modern Herbals Trapped Wind and Indigestion Tablets | for flatulence, indigestion and heartburn including dyspepsia and occasional diarrhoea | charcoal |
| Potter's Acidosis Tablets | for indigestion, stomach ache, heartburn and acid stomach | meadowsweet, rhubarb, vegetable charcoal |
| – Acidosis Mixture | indigestion, heartburn, flatulence | meadowsweet, gentian, euonymus |
| – Appetiser Mixture | to promote appetite and relieve flatulence | camomile, calumba, gentian |
| – Indian Brandee | for digestive discomfort and mild colic | capsicum, ginger, rhubarb |
| – Indigestion Mixture | for indigestion, heartburn, flatulence | meadowsweet, gentian, euonymus |
| – Pegina | for indigestion and flatulence | calumba, sweet flag, cardamom, magnesium sulphate, magnesium trisilicate, rhubarb and herbal oils |
| – Slippery Elm | for indigestion and flatulence | slippery elm, peppermint, anise, cinnamon |
| – Stomach Mixture | for stomach ache and stomach upsets | bismuth ammonium citrate, dandelion, gentian, rhubarb |
| Weleda Carminative Tea | for flatulence | aniseed, caraway, yarrow, matricaria |

| Products | Uses | Ingredients |
|----------|------|-------------|

## Homoeopathic

| | | |
|----------|------|-------------|
| argent nit | for upset, rumbling stomach due to apprehension | silver nitrate |
| arsen alb | for lack of appetite and weakness after illness | arsenic trioxide |
| berberis | for gallstones | berberis |
| bryonia | for indigestion straight after eating, colic | bryony |
| carbo veg | for a stomach full of wind | vegetable charcoal |
| chamomilla | for colic | chamomile |
| china | for gallstones | cinchona |
| colocynthis | for flatulence with colicky stomach pain | bitter cucumber |
| lycopodium | for indigestion from starchy food, wind, heartburn | club moss |
| nux vom | for indigestion from overindulgence | nux vomica |
| pulsatilla | for indigestion from rich foods | pasque flower |

New Era Tissue Salts:

| | | |
|----------|------|-------------|
| – No. 2 Calc Phos | for impaired digestion | calcium phosphate |
| – No. 8 Mag Phos | for flatulence | magnesium phosphate |
| – No. 10 Nat Phos | for gastric disorders, heartburn | sodium phosphate |
| – No. 11 Nat Sulph | for liverish symptoms, bilious attacks | sodium sulphate |
| – Combination C | for acidity, heartburn, dyspepsia | magnesium phosphate, sodium sulphate, silicon dioxide |
| – Combination E | for indigestion, colicky pain and flatulence | calcium phosphate, magnesium phosphate, sodium phosphate, sodium sulphate |
| – Combination S | for stomach upsets, biliousness | potassium chloride, sodium phosphate, sodium sulphate |

| Products | Uses | Ingredients |
|---|---|---|

## Anthroposophical

Wala Pillules
- Belladonna/Chamomilla — for relief of stomach aches and cramps — belladonna, matricaria

Weleda
- Digestodoron Tablets and Drops — for relief of indigestion — male fern, polypodium, willow, hart's tongue
- Carbo Betulae 3x Tablets — for relief of flatulence — charcoal
- Carvon Tablets — for relief of indigestion with flatulence — charcoal, oleum aetherium
- Choleodoron Drops — for gall bladder problems — celandine, turmeric
- Fragaria/Vitis Tablets — for relief of bilious symptoms and nervous indigestion — wild strawberry, grape vine

## Allopathic

| Products | Uses | Ingredients |
|---|---|---|
| Aluminium Hydroxide Mixture BP | for relief of indigestion and heartburn | aluminium hydroxide |
| Magnesium Trisilicate Mixture BP | for relief of indigestion, heartburn and dyspepsia | magnesium trisilicate, magnesium carbonate, sodium bicarbonate |
| Acidex | for heartburn (including in pregnancy), dyspepsia | sodium bicarbonate, sodium alginate, calcium carbonate |
| Actonorm Powder carbonate, | for hyperacidity, flatulence, dyspepsia, indigestion due to overeating | aluminium hydroxide, atropine, calcium magnesium carbonate, magnesium trisilicate, peppermint, sodium bicarbonate |
| Algicon Suspension and Tablets | heartburn associated with reflux and pregnancy and hyperacidity | magnesium alginate, aluminium hydroxide – magnesium carbonate cogel, magnesium carbonate, potassium bicarbonate |
| Alu-cap | for excess acid | aluminium hydroxide |
| Aludrox Liquid and Tablets | for indigestion, excess acidity | aluminium hydroxide |

| Products | Uses | Ingredients |
|---|---|---|
| Andrews<br>– Antacid | for heartburn, acid indigestion and trapped wind | calcium carbonate, magnesium carbonate |
| – Original Salts | for indigestion, overindulgence and constipation | sodium bicarbonate, citric acid, magnesium sulphate |
| Atkinson and Barkers Infant Gripe Mixture | for relief of griping pains and wind in babies | dill, caraway |
| Birley's Antacid Powder | for indigestion, stomach acidity, flatulence biliousness, heartburn | aluminium hydroxide, magnesium trisilicate, magnesium carbonate |
| Bisodol Indigestion Relief Powder and Tablets | for indigestion, dyspepsia, heartburn, acidity and flatulence | calcium carbonate, magnesium carbonate, sodium bicarbonate |
| Bragg's Medicinal Charcoal Tablets and Biscuits | for indigestion, wind and heartburn | vegetable charcoal |
| Buscopan | for irritable bowel syndrome, cramps | hyoscine |
| Carbellon | for indigestion, flatulence, dyspepsia | charcoal, magnesium hydroxide |
| Colpermin | for relief of irritable bowel syndrome | peppermint |
| De Witt's Antacid Powder and Tablets | for indigestion, gastric acidity, dyspepsia, heartburn and stomach discomfort | calcium carbonate, magnesium carbonate, magnesium trisilicate, peppermint |
| Eno | for indigestion, flatulence and nausea | sodium bicarbonate, citric acid, sodium carbonate |
| Equilon Herbal | for relief of irritable bowel syndrome | peppermint |
| Gastrocote Liquid and Tablets | for relief of acid indigestion and heartburn | sodium alginate, aluminium hydroxide, magnesium trisilicate, sodium bicarbonate |
| Gaviscon – Liquid | for heartburn and associated indigestion | sodium alginate, sodium bicarbonate, calcium carbonate |

| Products | Uses | Ingredients |
| --- | --- | --- |
| – Tablets | for heartburn and associated indigestion | alginic acid, sodium bicarbonate, aluminium hydroxide, magnesium trisilicate |
| – Advance | for gastric reflux, reflux oesophagitis, flatulence, heartburn, hiatus hernia | sodium alginate, potassium bicarbonate |
| – Infant | for gastric regurgitation, gastro-oesophageal reflux in infants and young children | sodium alginate, magnesium alginate |
| Jackson's Indian Brandee | for flatulence and digestive discomfort | cardamom, capsicum |
| Maalox Suspension | for gastritis, hyperacidity, heartburn | aluminium hydroxide, magnesium hydroxide |
| Milk of Magnesia | for upset stomach, indigestion, heartburn | magnesium hydroxide |
| Mintec | for relief of irritable bowel, spastic colon | peppermint |
| Nurse Harvey's Gripe Mixture | for wind, griping pains, stomach upsets | sodium bicarbonate, dill, caraway |
| Opas Tablets | for acid indigestion, heartburn, flatulence and dyspepsia | sodium bicarbonate, magnesium carbonate, calcium carbonate, magnesium trisilicate |
| Rap-eze | for indigestion and heartburn | calcium carbonate |
| Remegel | for indigestion and heartburn | calcium carbonate |
| Rennie | for indigestion, heartburn, flatulence, acidity and dyspepsia | calcium carbonate, magnesium carbonate |
| Rennie Duo | for heartburn and acid indigestion – may be used in pregnancy | calcium carbonate, sodium alginate |
| Setlers Antacid Tablets | for indigestion, heartburn, flatulence | calcium carbonate |

| Products | Uses | Ingredients |
|----------|------|-------------|
| Topal Tablets | for heartburn and discomfort due to reflux, oesophagitis, hiatus hernia, gastritis | alginic acid, aluminium hydroxide, magnesium carbonate |
| Tums | for acid indigestion, heartburn, flatulence | calcium carbonate |
| Woodward's Gripe Mixture | for relief of distress due to wind | dill, sodium bicarbonate |

# Mouth - Ulcers, Cold Sores, Toothache

Mouth ulcers are extremely common and can be due to a variety of causes such as vitamin deficiency, ill-fitting dentures or hormonal problems.

Toothache indicates a problem that needs a visit to the dentist as the products available only give temporary relief.

Some medicines cause dry mouth as a side effect which can be alleviated with saliva substitutes, available to buy or on prescription.

Cold sores are caused by a virus which everyone has around their mouth. No-one knows why some people get lots of cold sores and others never do. The virus is highly contagious and can be spread by kissing or touching the lips with the fingers. Cold sores are not just a winter complaint as bright sunlight can trigger an attack as well.

| Products | Uses | Ingredients |
|---|---|---|
| **Homoeopathic** | | |
| aconite | for toothache with shooting pains | aconite |
| arnica | for pain after a filling or extraction | arnica |
| arsen alb | for mouth ulcers, mouth dry and hot | arsenic trioxide |
| calc fluor | for toothache associated with bad dentition | calcium fluoride |
| cantharis | for mouth ulcers due to burning mouth with hot food | spanish fly |
| coffea | for toothache made worse by heat or pressure | coffee |
| merc sol | for toothache worse at night or from drinks | |
| nat mur | for mouth ulcers due to stress | sodium chloride |
| New Era Tissue Salts: | | |
| – No. 2 Calc Phos | for teething troubles | calcium phosphate |
| – No. 3 Calc Sulph | for sore lips | calcium sulphate |

| Products | Uses | Ingredients |
|---|---|---|

## Anthroposophical

| | | |
|---|---|---|
| Welda Medicinal Gargle | for mouth ulcers and oral hygiene | rhatany, myrrh, clove, sage, eucalyptus, rosegeranium, lavender, peppermint, horse chestnut, silver nitrate, calcium fluoride, magnesium sulphate |

## Allopathic

| | | |
|---|---|---|
| Clove Oil BP | for temporary relief of toothache | clove |
| Compound Thymol Glycerin Mouthwash BP | for oral hygiene | glycerol, thymol |
| Betadine Gargle and Mouthwash | for bacterial, fungal and viral mouth and throat infections; for dental surgery | iodine |
| Colsor Cream and Lotion | for cold sores | tannic acid, phenol, menthol |
| Dentogen | | |
| – Gel | temporary relief of toothache | clove |
| – Clove Oil Liquid | temporary relief of toothache | clove |
| Frador | for mouth ulcers and sores | menthol, chlorbutol, storax, benzoin |
| Pyralvex | for pain of mouth ulcers, denture irritation | anthroquinone glycosides of rhubarb, salicylic acid |

# Nausea and Travel Sickness

Travel sickness is miserable for those who suffer from it. The symptoms include nausea, dizziness, vomiting, sweating and increased saliva production. These symptoms can be reduced by avoiding large meals, especially greasy or spicy ones, and alcohol, both before and during journeys. It helps if sufferers avoid trying to read and instead look at the view in the distance. On board ships, staying in the centre of the vessel and looking at the horizon will help. Travel sickness remedies should be taken before the start of the journey for best relief. Ginger is a safe natural remedy, even in pregnancy.

Preparations containing hyoscine should not be taken by those with glaucoma and should be used with caution by those with urinary problems, high blood pressure and heart disease.

| Products | Uses | Ingredients |
|---|---|---|
| **Herbal** | | |
| Gerard House Ginger Tablets | carminative | ginger |
| Weleda Melissa Comp. | for nausea, stomach ache, stomach upsets and occasional diarrhoea | lemon balm, nutmeg, cinnamon, angelica, lemon oil, coriander, clove |
| **Homoeopathic** | | |
| arsen alb | for diarrhoea and vomiting | arsenic trioxide |
| cocculus | for travel sickness | indian cockle |
| ipecac | for persistent nausea and griping pains | ipecacuanha |
| nux vom | for vomiting 2–3 hours after eating, with retching | nux vomica |
| phosphorus | for vomiting as soon as food is warmed by stomach | phosphoric acid |
| pulsatilla | for vomiting after rich, fatty foods | pasque flower |

| Products | Uses | Ingredients |
|---|---|---|
| Nelson's Travella | travel sickness | apomorph, staphisagria, cocculus, theridion, petroleum, tabacum, nux vomica |

## Anthroposophical

| Wala Pillles | | |
|---|---|---|
| – Aurum/Valeriana | for nausea and dizziness of travel sickness | gold, valerian |

## Allopathic

| Joy-Rides | for the prevention of travel sickness | hyoscine |
|---|---|---|
| Kwells & Kwells Junior | for the prevention of travel sickness | hyoscine |

# Pain – Oral Preparations

More pain-killing tablets are sold than any other category of medicine, mainly aspirin, paracetamol and ibuprofen (which are not of natural origin), sometimes in combination with codeine and caffeine, which are both of natural origin. The products listed below are all of natural origin and are extremely safe, with few side effects. However, these products should not be taken during pregancy or while breast-feeding, except raspberry leaf, which should be taken during the last two weeks and during labour. Products containing kelp or bladderwrack should not be taken by those with thyroid disorders.

These products are not recommended for children.

| Products | Uses | Ingredients |
|---|---|---|
| **Herbal** | | |
| Bio-Strath Willow Formula | for relief of backache, lumbago, sciatica, fibrositis and muscular pain | willow, primula, yeast |
| Dorwest Kelp Seaweed Tablets | rheumatism, obesity | kelp |
| Mixed Vegetable Tablets | for rheumatism, cystitis and minor bladder conditions | watercress, celery, horseradish, parsley |
| Gerard House Kelp Tablets | for rheumatic pain and obesity | kelp |
| Reumalex | for rheumatic aches and pains, fibrositis, lumbago, backache and stiffness | lignum vitae, black cohosh, white willow, sarsaparilla, poplar |
| Heath and Heather Raspberry Leaf Tablets | for pain in chidbirth | raspberry leaf |
| Herbal Concepts – Backache Relief | for relief of backache | buchu, bearberry, parsley piert |
| – Daily Menopause Relief | for minor conditions associated with the menopause | lime, motherwort, pasque flower, valerian |
| – Period Pain Relief | for premenstrual tension and period pain | lady's mantle, motherwort, valerian, pasque flower, vervain, false unicorn |

# P

| Products | Uses | Ingredients |
|---|---|---|
| – Rheumatic Pain Relief | for rheumatic aches and pains | bogbean, lignum vitae, capsicum, celery |
| Hofels White Willow and Burdock | for symptomatic relief of rheumatic pain | white willow, burdock, prickly ash, bearberry, poplar |
| Lane's Vegetex Tablets | for muscular rheumatic pain, lumbago, and fibrositis | celery, buckbean, black cohosh |
| Modern Herbals Rheumatic Pain Tablets | for muscular rheumatic pain, lumbago, and fibrositis | celery, buckbean, black cohosh |
| Potter's<br>– Anased | for minor aches especially when associated with tension | hops |
| – Backache Tablets | for backache | gravel root, hydrangea, buchu, bearberry |
| – Backache Mixture | for backache | bearberry, juniper, clivers, dandelion, burdock |
| – Black Haw and Golden Seal Elixir | for relief of discomfort in middle-of-life women | black haw, golden seal |
| – Raspberry Leaf | for menstrual pain | raspberry |
| – Rheumatic Pain | for relief of rheumatic aches and pains | bogbean, burdock, yarrow, lignum vitae, nutmeg |
| – Sciargo | for sciatica and lumbago | juniper, wild carrot, shepherd's purse, clivers, bearberry |
| – St John's wort Compound | for sciatica | juniper, st john's wort, white willow, black cohosh, scullcap |
| – Tabritis | rheumatic pain and stiffness, maintains joint mobility | elder, yarrow, prickly ash, burdock, clivers, poplar, senna, bearberry |
| – Willow Bark Tablets | for any condition where a herb derived salicylate is needed | white willow |
| Rheumasol | for muscular pain and stiffness associated with backache, sciatica, lumbago, fibrositis | lignum vitae, prickly ash |

| Products | Uses | Ingredients |
|----------|------|-------------|

## Homoeopathic

| Products | Uses | Ingredients |
|----------|------|-------------|
| actaea rac | for muscular soreness and bruising, painful periods | black cohosh |
| aconite | for fibrositis | aconite |
| apis mel | for burning stinging pains | honey-bee |
| arnica | for pains due to bruising | arnica |
| belladonna | for pain worse before period | belladonna |
| bryonia | for pain worse on movement, headaches | bryony |
| chamomilla | for cramping period pains | chamomile |
| cuprum met | for severe cramps in feet and legs | copper metal |
| euphrasia | for headache with watery eyes | eyebright |
| gelsemium | for headache and pain when period late and scanty | gelsemium |
| hypericum | for headache and migraine | st john's wort |
| ignatia | for piercing frontal or temporal hammering | st ignatius's bean |
| kali bich | for migraine preceded by blurred vision | potassium bichromate |
| kali phos | for headache of migraine with humming in the ears | potassium phosphate |
| ledum | for fibrositis | marsh tea |
| lycopodium | for headache on right side | club moss |
| nat mur | for throbbing, blinding headache and migraine | sodium chloride |
| nux vom | for prolonged period which comes early | nux vomica |
| pulsatilla | for pain in joints, headaches | pasque flower |
| rhus tox | for pain worse on starting to move, which improves on movement | poison ivy |
| ruta grav | for painful joints | rue |

| Products | Uses | Ingredients |
|---|---|---|
| silicea | for migraine which travels over head to eye | silicon dioxide |
| thuja | for left-sided headache | white cedar |
| Nelson's | | |
| – Rheumatica | for rheumatic pain | poison oak |
| – Teetha | for teething | white bryony |
| New Era Tissue Salts: | | |
| – No. 8 Mag Phos | for cramp, neuralgia, nerve pains | magnesium phosphate |
| – No. 10 Nat Phos | for rheumatic tendency | sodium phosphate |
| – Combination A | for sciatica, neuralgia, neuritis | iron phosphate, potassium phosphate, magnesium phosphate |
| – Combination F | for migraine, nervous headache | potassium phosphate, magnesium phosphate, sodium chloride, silicon dioxide |
| – Combination G | for backache, lumbago, piles | calcium fluoride, calcium phosphate, potassium phosphate, sodium chloride |
| – Combination I | for fibrositis and muscular pain | iron phosphate, potassium sulphate, magnesium phosphate |
| – Combination L | for varicose veins, circulatory disorders | calcium fluoride, iron phosphate, sodium chloride |
| – Combination M | for rheumatism | calcium phosphate, potassium chloride, sodium phosphate, sodium sulphate |
| – Combination N | for menstrual pain | calcium phosphate, potassium chloride, potassium phosphate, magnesium phosphate |
| – Combination P | for aching feet and legs | calcium fluoride, calcium phosphate, potassium phosphate, magnesium phosphate |

| Products | Uses | Ingredients |
|---|---|---|
| – Combination R | for infants' teething pains | calcium fluoride, calcium phosphate, iron phosphate, magnesium phosphate, silicon dioxide |
| – Combination S | for sick headache | potassium chloride, sodium phosphate, sodium sulphate |
| – Elasto Tablets | for relief of aching legs | calcium fluoride, calcium phosphate, iron phosphate, magnesium phosphate |

## Anthroposophical

Wala Pillules

| | | |
|---|---|---|
| – Apis/Bryonia | for muscular rheumatic pain, lumbago | honey-bee, white bryony |
| – Apis/Levisticum | for relief of sciatica | honey-bee, lovage |
| – Chamomilla/Nicotiana | for relief of period pains | matricaria, nicotiana |
| – Magnesium Phosphoricum | for muscular cramps and stiff muscles | magnesium phosphate |
| – Sanguinaria comp. | for headaches and migraine | bloodroot |

Weleda Bidor

| | | |
|---|---|---|
| – 1% Tablets | for prevention and relief of migraine | ferrous sulphate, silica |
| – 5% Tablets | for symptomatic relief of migraine | ferrous sulphate, silica |
| – Chamomilla 3x Pillules | for relief of teething and colic | german chamomile |
| – Mandragora Comp. Drop | for relief of arthritic rheumatic pain | arnica, birch, horsetail, mandrake, meniscus |
| – Menodoron Drops | for relief of irregularities of the menstrual cycle including painful periods | shepherd's purse, marjoram, yarrow, oak, nettle |
| – Rheumadoron 102A Drops | for relief of muscular and rheumatic pain | aconite, arnica, birch, mandrake |
| – Rheumadoron 1 Drop | for relief of rheumatic pain | aconite, arnica, bryony |
| – Rheumadoron 2 Drops | for relief of rheumatic pain | meadow saffron, savine |

| Products | Uses | Ingredients |
|---|---|---|
| **Allopathic** | | |
| Ashton and Parson's Infant Powders | for relief of pain and gastric upset associated with teething | matricaria |
| Crampex Tablets | for prevention of night muscle cramps | nicotinic acid, cholecalc-iferol, calcium gluconate |
| Seven Seas – Pure Cod-Liver Oil | for relief of joint pains and stiffness | cod-liver oil |
| – Orange Syrup and Cod-Liver Oil + extra vitamins | for relief of joint pains and stiffness | cod-liver oil, vitamins, orange |

## Pain – Topical Preparations

The products listed in this section are indicated for muscular and rheumatic pain, such as fibrositis, sciatica, lumbago, sprains, strains, bruising and stiffness and unbroken chilblains. Many contain salicylates (a mild topical counterirritant and analgesic), and volatile oils, which cause local vasodilatation and mild analgesia. Capsicum is a strong counterirritant. It is important that these products are not applied to broken skin.

| Products | Uses | Ingredients |
|---|---|---|
| **Herbal** | | |
| Lane's Gonne Rheumatic Balm | for muscular pains and stiffness | camphor, menthol, eucalyptus, methyl salicylate, turpentine |
| Modern Herbals Muscular Pain Cream | for muscular pains and stiffness | camphor, menthol, eucalyptus, methyl salicylate, turpentine |
| Potter's Nine Rubbing Oils | for muscular pain and stiffness, backache, lumbago, sciatica, fibrositis, rheumatic pain and strains | amber, clove, eucalyptus, linseed, methyl salicylate, mustard, thyme, turpentine, peppermint, arachis |

| Products | Uses | Ingredients |
|---|---|---|
| Weleda | | |
| – Arnica Massage Balm | rheumatic pain, muscular pain, and stiffness | sunflower, arnica, birch, rosemary, lavender |
| – Massage Balm with Calendula | rheumatic and muscular pain, stiffness, backache, fibrositis, bruising, sprains | marigold |

## Homoeopathic

| | | |
|---|---|---|
| Nelson's | | |
| – Rhus Tox Cream | for rheumatic conditions, pain, strains | poison oak |
| – Strains Ointment | for bruised bone, strained tendons | rue |

## Anthroposophical

| | | |
|---|---|---|
| Weleda | | |
| – Copper Ointment | for relief of muscular pain and cramps | copper |
| – Rheumadoron Ointment | for relief of muscular rheumatic pain | aconite, arnica, birch, mandrake, rosemary |
| – Rhus Tox Ointment | for relief of rheumatic pain and stiffness | poison oak |
| – Ruta Ointment | for relief of sprains and dislocations | rue |
| – Skin Tone Lotion | to refresh and revitalise tired limbs | citrus medica, arnica, burdock, blackthorn, iris, prunus, witch hazel, lemon, tragacanth, glycerol, copper sulphate, sodium silicate, citric acid |

## Allopathic

| | | |
|---|---|---|
| Eucalyptus Oil BP | for muscular sprains and cramps | eucalyptus |
| Wintergreen Ointment BP | for relief of pain in lumbago, sciatica and rheumatism | methyl salicylate |
| Algipan | for relief of muscular and rheumatic pain | methyl nicotinate, glycol salicylate, capsicum |

| Products | Uses | Ingredients |
|---|---|---|
| Avoca Menthol Cone | for relief of headaches | menthol |
| Balmosa | for pain associated with chilblains, muscular rheumatism, fibrositis, lumbago | menthol, camphor, methyl salicylate, capsicum |
| Chymol Emollient Balm | for chapped and sore skin, chilblains bruises and sprains | eucalyptus, terpineol, methyl salicylate, phenol |
| Cremalgin | for muscular pain, stiffness, lumbago, rheumatism, sciatica, fibrositis | methyl nicotinate, capsicum, glycol monosalicylate |
| Cuxson Gerrard Belladonna Plaster | for lumbago, rheumatism, sciatica, muscular tension, backache, stiff neck | belladonna |
| Deep Freeze | | |
| – Spray | for muscular pain and stiffness | menthol |
| – Cold Gel | for pain of joints, muscles, tendons | menthol |
| Deep Heat | | |
| – Maximum Strength | for muscular pain and stiffness, backache, lumbago, sciatica, fibrositis, sprains | methyl salicylate, menthol |
| – Massage Liniment | bruises, rheumatic pain | methyl salicylate, menthol |
| – Rub | | methyl salicylate, menthol, eucalyptus, turpentine |
| – Spray | | methyl nicotinate and salicylates |
| Dubam | | |
| – Spray | for muscular pain and stiffness | methyl nicotinate and salicylates |
| – Cream | for muscular pain and stiffness | methyl salicylate, menthol, cineole |
| Ellimans Embrocation | for muscular pains and stiffness | turpentine, acetic acid |
| Fiery Jack – Ointment | for sciatica, lumbago, fibrositis, rheumatic | capsicum |

| Products | Uses | Ingredients |
|---|---|---|
| – Cream | pain, muscular pain, stiffness | capsicum, methyl nicotinate, glycol and diethylamine salicylate |
| Goddard's Emulsion | for muscular pain and stiffness | turpentine, acetic acid, ammonia |
| 4Head | natural headache relief | levomenthol |
| Hansaplast Thermo | for muscular and rheumatic pain | capsicum, arnica |
| Nasciodine | for rheumatic pain, strains, bruises, chilblains | iodine, menthol, methyl salicylate, turpentine, camphor |
| PR Heat Spray | for muscular pain and stiffness | methyl salicylate, ethyl nicotinate, camphor |
| Quool | for relief of muscular discomfort | menthol |
| Radian-B<br>– Muscle Lotion and Pump Action Spray | for muscular pain and stiffness | menthol, camphor, ammonium salicylate, salicylic acid |
| – Muscle Rub | for relief of muscular and rheumatic pain | menthol, camphor, methyl salicylate, capsicum |
| Ralgex<br>– Cream<br>– Heat Spray<br>– Stick | for muscular aches and stiffness | methyl nicotinate, capsicum, glycol monosalicylate, salicylates, capsicum, menthol |
| Salonair | for muscular pain and stiffness | methyl salicylate, menthol, camphor, benzyl nicotinate, squalene, glycol salicylate |
| Salonpas Plasters | for muscular pain and joint aches | salicylates |
| Tiger Balm Red and White | for minor muscular aches and pains | camphor, menthol, cajuput, clove |
| Vadarex | for muscular aches and pains | methyl salicylate, menthol |

# Skin – Acne, Eczema, Psoriasis, Damaged Skin and Nappy Rash

Emollients soothe and soften dry skin. They can be applied directly to dry or wet skin or used as a bath additive. If used in the bath take care when you get out as these products can make the bath very slippery.

Dermatitis and eczema both exhibit an inflammatory response with red scaly eruptions; eczema, which is a chronic allergic disorder, is often associated with hay fever and asthma. Contact dermatitis is caused by an allergic response to a specific thing, such as nickel, detergents, wool, perfume, even insect bites, with the inflammatory response only affecting the area in contact with the cause.

Psoriasis is a chronic scaly skin disorder which often runs in families. In psoriasis new skin cells are produced about 10 times faster than normal. This results in thickened patches covered with dead, flaking skin. The affected area can be quite extensive and causes great physical discomfort and social embarrassment. Treament is with emollients and coal-tar products.

Ichthyosis is a rare, inherited condition in which the skin is dry, thickened, scaly and darker than normal due to an abnormality in the production of keratin (a protein which is a major component of skin). Treatment is with emollients; soap needs to be avoided.

Xeroderma pigmentosum is another rare, inherited skin disease in which the skin, due to photosensitivity, becomes prematurely aged, and skin cancers can develop. Treatment is by wearing protective clothing, sunscreens and emollients.

Acne is a chronic skin disorder caused by inflammation of the hair follicles and the sebaceous glands of the skin. There is no instant cure for acne; excessive washing will not help. Blackheads are nothing to do with not washing: they are caused by the natural oils produced by the skin blocking the sebaceous glands and becoming oxidised, which changes the colour to black. Some people find that creams by themselves are not effective, and have to seek help from their doctor, who can prescribe a six-month course of antibiotics or one of the skin preparations based on vitamin A.

Nappy rash is a form of dermatitis, caused by ammonia on the wet nappy being in contact with the skin, by allergy to detergents, or by

bacterial or fungal infections. Since the introduction of disposable
nappies and the improvements made to them, nappy rash is far less
common than in the past. Nappies should be changed as soon after
soiling as possible with the area washed and carefully dried before
putting on a new nappy. Waterproof pants should be avoided.

| Products | Uses | Ingredients |
|---|---|---|
| **Herbal** | | |
| Gerard House – Echinacea Tablets | minor skin conditions, acne, mild eczema | echinacea |
| – Skin | for spots, skin blemishes and dry eczema | burdock, wild pansy |
| Heath and Heather Skin Tablets | for spots, skin blemishes and dry eczema | burdock, wild pansy |
| HRI Clear Complexion | to help minor skin conditions and acne | sarsaparilla, blue flag, burdock |
| Lane's Tea Tree and Witch Hazel Cream | for minor skin conditions, dry, chapped skin, nappy rash, minor burns and sunburn | eucalyptus, camphor, witch hazel, methyl salicylate, zinc oxide, tea tree |
| Potter's – Echinacea Elixir | for minor skin conditions and catarrh | echinacea, wild indigo, fumitory |
| – Echinacea Tablets | for skin conditions and blemishes | echinacea |
| – Eczema Ointment | for eczema | zinc oxide, salicylic acid, benzoic acid, chickweed, lanolin |
| – Herbheal Ointment | for skin conditions where there is irritation | colophony, starch, sulphur, zinc oxide, marshmallow, chickweed |
| – Jamaican Sarsaparilla Liquid | minor skin complaints and rashes | sarsaparilla, capsicum, glycerin, liquorice, peppermint, treacle |
| – Psorasolv Ointment | for mild psoriasis | starch, sulphur, zinc oxide, poke root, clivers |
| – Skin Clear | for skin conditions and blemishes | echinacea |

| Products | Uses | Ingredients |
|----------|------|-------------|
| – Skin Clear Ointment | for mild eczema and difficult skin conditions | starch, sulphur, zinc oxide, tea tree |
| – Skin Eruptions Mixture | mild eczema, psoriasis, and other skin diseases | blue flag, burdock, yellow dock, sarsaparilla, buchu, cascara |
| – Varicose Ointment | for irritating skin conditions due to varicosity | cade oil, witch hazel, zinc oxide |

## Homoeopathic

| | | |
|----------|------|-------------|
| arsen alb | for psoriasis and boils | arsenic trioxide |
| belladonna | for acne and boils | belladonna |
| calc carb | for nappy rash and chilblains | calcium carbonate |
| graphites | for eczema on hands and behind ears | graphite |
| hepar sulph | for eczema of sensitive skin, acne and boils | calcium sulphide |
| nat mur | for oily skin with many little pimples | sodium chloride |
| pulsatilla | for spots made worse by rich fatty food, chilblains | pasque flower |
| rhus tox | for itchy eczema, acne and nappy rash | poison ivy |
| silicea | for acne and boils where skin scars easily | silicon dioxide |
| sulphur | for dry eczema, psoriasis, acne and nappy rash | sulphur |
| Bach Rescue Cream | to soothe and restore skin | cherry plum, clematis, crab apple, impatiens, rock rose, star of bethlehem |

Nelson's

| | | |
|----------|------|-------------|
| – Calendula Cream | for rough and sore skin | marigold |
| – Chilblains Ointment | for chilblains | black bryony |
| – Evening Primrose Cream | for dry tired skin | evening primrose |
| – Graphites Cream | for dermatitis | graphites |

| Products | Uses | Ingredients |
|---|---|---|
| – Healing Ointment | promotes rapid, safe healing of cuts, sores, abrasions, rough, sore, sensitive skin | marigold |
| – Hypercal Cream | for cuts and sores | marigold, st john's wort |

New Era
Tissue Salts:

| | | |
|---|---|---|
| – No. 3 Calc Sulph | for acne, pimples, skin slow to heal | calcium sulphate |
| – No. 7 Kali Sulph | for maintaining skin condition and skin eruptions with scaling and exudations | potassium sulphate |
| – No. 12 Silica | for boils, brittle nails | silicon dioxide |
| – Combination D | for minor skin ailments | calcium sulphate, potassium chloride, potassium sulphate, silicon dioxide |

## Anthroposophical

| | | |
|---|---|---|
| Wala Pillules – Urtica comp. | for pruritis, eczema, dermatitis | nettle |

Weleda

| | | |
|---|---|---|
| – Balsamicum Ointment | for nappy rash | marigold, dog's mercury, peru balsam, antimony |
| – Dermatodoron Ointment | for eczema | bittersweet, loosestrife |
| – Dulcamara/ Lysmachia Drops | for relief of eczema | bittersweet, loosestrife |
| – Frost Cream | for chilblains | abrotanum, arnica, peru balsam, rosemary, antimony |
| – WCS Dusting Powder | for minor burns, soreness and slow-healing wounds | arnica, marigold, echinacea, antimony, purified talc. |

## Allopathic

| | | |
|---|---|---|
| Aqueous Cream BP | a skin cleanser and emollient | water, emulsifying wax |
| Calamine Aqueous Cream BP | for itching | calamine, zinc oxide, liquid paraffin |
| Emulsifying Ointment BP | a soap substitute and emollient | white soft and liquid paraffin, emulsifying wax |

| Products | Uses | Ingredients |
|---|---|---|
| Friar's Balsam BP | for use as an antiseptic and inhalant | storax, benzoin, aloes |
| Glycerin BP | for rough, chapped skin and sore throats | glycerin |
| Hydrous Ointment BP | emollient | magnesium sulphate, wool alcohols, water |
| Magnesium Sulphate Paste BP | a drawing ointment for boils | magnesium sulphate, glycerol, phenol |
| White Soft Paraffin BP | emollient | paraffin, white soft |
| Yellow Soft Paraffin BP | emollient | paraffin, yellow soft |
| Zinc and Castor Oil Ointment BP | for nappy and urinary rash | zinc oxide, castor oil, arachis oil, beeswax |
| Zinc and Salicylic Acid (Lassar's) Paste BP | for hyperkeratotic skin disorders | zinc oxide, salicylic acid, starch, white soft paraffin |
| Acnisal | for mild to moderate eczema | salicylic acid |
| Alcoderm Cream | for dry, chapped or irritated skin | liquid paraffin |
| Alpha Keri Bath Oil | for dry itchy skin, ichthyosis | mineral oil, lanolin oil |
| Alphosyl Cream and Lotion | for psoriasis | coal tar, allantoin |
| Antipeol | for minor skin problems | ichthammol, salicylic acid, urea |
| Aquadrate | for ichthyosis, xeroderma, hyperkeratosis | urea |
| Aveeno<br>– Cream | for eczema, xeroderma, ichthyosis | oatmeal |
| – Bath Oil | for eczema, xeroderma, ichthyosis | oatmeal |
| – Colloidal Bath Additive | for itchy problems like chickenpox | oatmeal |
| Balneum | for dry skin with dermatitis and eczema | soya oil |

| Products | Uses | Ingredients |
|----------|------|-------------|
| Calmurid | for hyperkeratosis, ichthyosis | urea, lactic acid |
| Carbo-Dome | for psoriasis | coal tar |
| Cetraben | for dry skin | white soft and liquid paraffin |
| Chymol Emollient Balm | for chapped sore skin, chilblains | eucalyptus, terpineol, methyl salicylate, phenol |
| Clinitar Cream | for psoriasis, chronic atopic eczema | coal tar |
| DDD Medicated Lotion | for spots, pimples and minor rashes | thymol, menthol, salicylic acid, methyl salicylate, glycerol |
| DDD Medicated Cream | for spots, cuts, grazes, skin problems | thymol, menthol, methyl salicylate, chlorbutol, titanium dioxide |
| Dermalo | bath emollient for dry skin conditions | liquid paraffin, wool alcohols |
| Dermamist | for eczema, ichthyosis, pruritis | white soft and liquid paraffin, coconut |
| Diprobase | for inflamed, damaged, dry skin | liquid and white soft paraffin |
| E45 Cream | for dry skin conditions | white soft and liquid paraffin, lanolin |
| Epaderm | a soap substitute and emollient | yellow soft and liquid paraffin, emulsifying wax |
| Eucerin Cream & Lotion | for atopic eczema, ichthyosis, xeroderma | urea |
| Exorex Lotion | for psoriasis of skin and scalp | coal tar |
| Fuller's Earth Cream | for soothing and protecting the skin | kaolin, zinc oxide, arachis oil, beeswax, paraffins |

| Products | Uses | Ingredients |
| --- | --- | --- |
| Gammaderm Cream | for symptomatic relief of acute and chronic dry skin conditions, restores hydration | evening primrose oil |
| Gelcosal | for psoriasis and chronic scaling dermatitis | coal tar, pine tar, salicylic acid |
| Gelcotar | for psoriasis and chronic dermatitis | coal tar, pine tar |
| Hewlett's Cream | for nappy rash, chapped and sore hands | zinc oxide, lanolin, oleic acid, arachis oil, rose oil, white soft paraffin |
| Imuderm Therapeutic Oil | for atopic eczema, dermatitis, pruritis | almond oil, liquid paraffin |
| Infaderm Theraputic Oil | for eczema, ichthyosis, psoriasis, pruritis | almond oil, liquid paraffin |
| Kamillosan | treatment of sore nipples in breast-feeding | chamomile |
| Keri Therapeutic Lotion | for nappy rash, dermatitis, eczema, ichthyosis | mineral oil |
| KL Kaolin Poultice | to draw boils | kaolin |
| KL Magnesium Sulphate | to draw boils | magnesium sulphate, glycerol |
| Melrose | for dry skin and chapped lips | yellow soft and liquid paraffin, lanolin, lemon grass |
| Morhulin | for eczema, nappy rash, minor wounds | zinc oxide, cod-liver oil |
| Neutrogena – Hand Cream | for dry skin conditions | glycerol |
| – Dermatological Cream | for dry skin conditions | glycerol |
| Nicam Gel | for mild to moderate inflammatory acne with papules and pustules | nicotinamide |
| Nostroline | soothes nostrils, nose and upper lip | menthol, eucalyptus, geranium |

| Products | Uses | Ingredients |
|---|---|---|
| Nutraplus Cream | for dry and damaged skin | urea |
| Oilatum – Bath Formula | for eczema, dermatitis, itchy conditions | liquid paraffin |
| – Cream | for eczema, dermatitis, itchy conditions | white soft and liquid paraffin |
| – Hand Aquagel | for eczema, dermatitis, itchy conditions | liquid paraffin |
| Papulex | for mild to moderate acne | nicotinamide |
| Snowfire | for chapped hands and chilblains | benzoin, citronella, thyme, lemon thyme, clove, cade oil |
| St James' Balm | for minor skin problems | zinc oxide, ichthammol, urea, salicylic acid |
| Ultrabase | for dry skin conditions | white soft and liquid paraffin |
| Vaseline | emollient | white soft paraffin |
| Witch Hazel – Distilled | a mild astringent and skin cleanser | witch hazel |

# Sleep

About 30% of the population suffers from sleep disturbance due to the stresses and strains of life. It is advisable, if you have a temporary sleep problem, to avoid alcohol, not sleep during the day, and to take some form of physical excercise.

These products are not suitable for children, in pregnancy or while breast-feeding.

| Products | Uses | Ingredients |
| --- | --- | --- |
| **Herbal** | | |
| Bio-Strath Valerian Formula | for relief of tenseness and irritability and to help promote natural sleep | valerian, passion flower, peppermint, yeast |
| Dorwest Scullcap and Gentian Tablets | irritability, sleeplessness, anxiety | scullcap, valerian, vervain, gentian |
| Gerard House Somnus | for relief of restlessness and to promote relaxation and sleep | valerian, hops, wild lettuce |
| Goodnight | for relief of sleeplessness and to promote natural sleep | vervain, hops, valerian, wild lettuce, passiflora |
| Heath and Heather Quiet Night Tablets | soothes and so aids natural sleep | valerian, hops, passion flower |
| Hofels Passiflora and Wild Lettuce | to promote natural sleep | passion flower, wild lettuce, hops, jamica dogwood |
| HRI Night | to promote natural sleep | valerian, passion flower, wild lettuce, vervain, hops |
| Lane's Naturest Tablets | temporary or occasional sleeplessness caused by secondary symptoms | passion flower |
| Modern Herbals Sleep Aid Passiflora Tablets | temporary or occasional sleeplessness caused by secondary symptoms | passion flower |
| Natrasleep | encourages natural sleep | hops, valerian |

| Products | Uses | Ingredients |
|---|---|---|
| Nytol Herbal | a herbal sleep aid | hops, jamaica dogwood, wild lettuce, passion flower, pasque flower |
| Phytocalm | to help relieve stress and strains of modern living and help promote sleep | passion flower |
| Potter's<br>– Nodoff Passiflora Tablets | aid to natural sleep | passion flower |
| – Nodoff Mixture | herbal sleeping draught | passion flower, scullcap, hops, valerian, jamaica dogwood |
| Sedonium | to promote natural sleep | valerian |
| Slumber Tablets | to promote natural sleep | wild lettuce, passion flower, hops, jamaica dogwood |
| Valerina Night-Time | to promote natural sleep | valerian, hops, lemon balm |

## Homoeopathic

| | | |
|---|---|---|
| aconite | for sleeplessness after shock or panic | aconite |
| arsen alb | for waking around midnight, restless, worried | arsenic trioxide |
| chamomilla | for children with teething and colic | chamomile |
| cocculus | for when you feel too tired to sleep | indian cockle |
| coffea | for sleeplessness with physical restlessness | coffee |
| ignatia | for sleeplessness due to upset or bereavement | st ignatius's bean |
| lycopodium | for when you can't switch off your mind | club moss |
| nux vom | when due to mental strain or overindulgence | nux vomica |
| pulsatilla | for when you feel too hot or cold in bed | pasque flower |
| rhus tox | when irritable and restless with pain and discomfort | poison oak |

| Products | Uses | Ingredients |
|---|---|---|
| Nelson's Noctura | insomnia and sleep difficulties | potassium bromide, coffee, passion flower, oats, alfalfa, valerian |

## Anthroposophical

Wala Pillules
– Valeriana Comp.          to aid peaceful relaxation     valerian
                           and natural sleep

# Slimming

The following products can aid slimming in conjunction with a calorie-controlled diet.

They are not recommended for patients with disorders of the thyroid gland.

They should not be taken in pregnancy or while breast-feeding.

They should not be taken by children.

| Product | Uses | Ingredients |
|---|---|---|
| **Herbal** | | |
| Adios | an aid to slimming | butternut, dandelion, boldo, bladderwrack |
| Boldo Aid to Slimming | to help weight loss | dandelion, boldo, bladderwrack |
| Dorwest Kelp Seaweed Tablets | rheumatism, obesity | kelp |
| Herbal Concepts Weight Loss Aid | aids weight reduction in conjunction with a calorie-controlled diet | dandelion, bladderwrack, boldo |
| Phytoslim | adjuvant to slimming diets | bladderwrack |
| Potter's Boldex Aid to Slimming | aid to slimming | boldo, butternut, dandelion, bladderwrack |

# Stress

The strains and stresses of modern life make us all tense and irritable at times.

Herbal, homoeopathic and anthroposophical remedies can offer a natural effective treatment.

These products are not recommended for children; some should not be taken in pregnancy or while breast-feeding. Some may cause drowsiness, in which case, if you are affected, avoid driving or operating machinery.

| Product | Uses | Ingredients |
| --- | --- | --- |
| **Herbal** | | |
| Dorwest Scullcap and Gentian Tablets | irritability, sleeplessness, anxiety | scullcap, valerian, vervain, gentian |
| Gerard House Serenity | irritability and life's stresses and strains | hops, passion flower, valerian |
| Heath and Heather Becalm Tablets | aids relaxation from everyday stresses | valerian, hops, passion flower |
| Herbal Concepts – Daily Tension and Strain Relief | relieves everyday tension and strain | asafetida, valerian, oats, passion flower |
| – Daily Fatigue Relief | for the alleviation of temporary fatigue and tiredness | kola, damiana, saw palmetto |
| – Daily Overwork and Mental Fatigue Relief | gentle aid to combat the effects of overwork | oats, prickly ash |
| Hofels Valerian and Gentian | for relief of tenseness and stress | valerian, gentian, scullcap, asafetida |
| HRI Calm Life | to help restlessness and irritability | jamaica dogwood, hops, scullcap, matricaria, valerian |
| Kalms | worry, irritability, exogenous stress and strain, also worry, wakefulness and other symptoms of the menopause including hot flushes and cold sweats; promotes sleep | hops, gentian, valerian |

| Products | Uses | Ingredients |
|---|---|---|
| Lane's Athera Tablets | for relief of minor conditions associated with the menopause | vervain, senna, clivers, parsley |
| Modern Herbals<br>– Menopause Tablets | for relief of minor conditions associated with the menopause | vervain, senna, clivers, parsley |
| – Stress Tablets | to reduce stresses, strains, irritabililty; aids restful sleep | motherwort, vervain, passion flower, valerian |
| Natracalm | for the stress and strain of everyday life | passion-flower |
| Phytocalm | to help relieve stress and strain and to promote natural sleep | passion-flower |
| Potter's<br>– Anased | for minor aches especially when associated with tension | hops |
| – Newrelax | tenseness, irritability, or agitation due to stresses and strains of modern life | hops, scullcap, valerian, vervain |
| – Prementaid | for mood-swing aggravation before periods | motherwort, pasque flower, bearberry, valerian |
| – Wellwoman | for the wellbeing of middle-aged (menopausal) women | yarrow, motherwort, lime flowers, scullcap, valerian |
| – Valerian Formula | for irritability and the stresses and strains of modern life | hops, scullcap, valerian, vervain |
| Quiet Life Tablets | to relieve periods of worry, irritability and exogenous stresses and strains and to promote natural sleep | hops, wild lettuce, valerian, motherwort, passion flower and B-group vitamins |
| Sedonium | to relieve stress and promote natural sleep | valerian |
| Stressless | for the stresses and strains of life | hops, scullcap, valerian, vervain |
| Valerina Daytime | for the stresses and strains of modern life | valerian, lemon balm |

| Products | Uses | Ingredients |
|---|---|---|

## Homoeopathic

| | | |
|---|---|---|
| aconite | for sudden panic attacks | aconite |
| argent nit | for fear of heights or crowds, lacking self-confidence | silver nitrate |
| arsen alb | feeling restless and irritable | arsenic trioxide |
| calc carb | for overwork and premenstrual tension | calcium carbonate |
| gelsemium | for exam nerves and fear of failure | gelsemium |
| ignatia | for anxiety following bereavement or breakup | st ignatius's bean |
| lycopodium | for anxiety about performing, stress of work | club moss |
| nat mur | for anxiety in those who don't like fuss and sympathy | sodium chloride |
| nux vom | for premenstrual tension, stress of work | nux vomica |
| phosphorus | for the highly nervous and sensitive | phosphoric acid |
| pulsatilla | for those who easily turn to tears | pasque flower |
| sepia | for women who are easily depressed, irritable and tearful, also hot flushes | sepia |
| New Era Tissue Salts: | | |
| – No. 6 Kali Phos | for nerve complaints and stress | potassium phosphate |
| – Combination B | for nervous exhaustion and general debility | calcium phosphate, iron phosphate, potassium phosphate |
| Bach Flower Remedies | for fear ...try | aspen, cherry plum, mimulus, red chestnut, rock rose |
| | for uncertainty ...try | cerato, gentian, gorse, hornbeam schleranthus, wild oat |
| | for lack of interest ...try | chestnut bud, clematis, honey-suckle, mustard, olive, white chestnut, wild rose |

| | | |
|---|---|---|
| | for loneliness ...try | heather, impatiens, water violet |
| | for oversensitivity to others ...try | agrimony, centaury, holly, walnut |
| | for over-concern for others ...try | beech, chicory, rock water, vervain, vine |
| | for despondency and despair ...try | crab apple, elm, larch, oak, pine, star of bethlehem, sweet chestnut, willow |
| Rescue Remedy | for emergencies to calm and balance and before stressful events | cherry plum, clematis, impatiens, rock rose, star of bethlehem |

## Anthroposophical

Wala Pillules

| | | |
|---|---|---|
| – Aurum/Prunus | for relief of exhaustion | gold, prunus |
| – Melissa/Sepia Comp. | for mild menopausal complaints, including hot flushes, irritability and exhaustion | lemon balm, sepia |
| – Meteoreisen/ Phosphor/Quartz | for relief of exhaustion from flu'-like symptoms | meteorite, phosphorus, silicon dioxide |

Weleda

| | | |
|---|---|---|
| – Avena Sativa Comp. | to aid relaxation | oats, hops, passion-flower valerian, coffee |
| – Fragador Tablets | for everyday stress and strain | scurvy grass, conchae, wild strawberry, glycogen, lovage, honey, chinese angelica, sage, wheatgerm, nettle, vivianite, sodium carbonate |

# Urinary Tract – Cystitis, Bladder, Water Balance

Cystitis is an inflammation of the bladder or urethra which can be caused by trauma or by a bacterial infection. It is very common in women, due to the short length of the urethra. However in men it is rare, because of the longer urethra, and usually occurs due to an obstruction, such as an enlarged prostate gland. Men with cystitis should always see their doctor for investigation and treatment. Failure of treatment with a purchased remedy means that an antibiotic prescribed by your doctor is necessary.

The bladder has a very complicated nerve supply, so defective bladder function can lead to problems such as incontinence or urinary retention from a variety of causes. The products listed may help but should not be taken for long periods of time.

Any continuing problems should be investigated by a doctor.

Water balance is a problem for many women in the week or so before their period; herbal remedies can be a great help in treating this.

Those with high blood pressure should avoid those allopathic remedies which contain sodium salts and choose potassium-containing remedies instead.

These products are not to be used by children and some are not to be used in pregnancy or whilst breast-feeding.

| Product | Uses | Ingredients |
|---|---|---|
| **Herbal** | | |
| Aqualette | for promotion of normal water balance | horsetail, dandelion |
| De Witts K and B Pills | for normal urinary elimination of water | bearberry, buchu |
| Dorwest Mixed Vegetable Tablets | for rheumatism, cystitis and minor bladder conditions | watercress, celery, horseradish, parsley |
| Gerard House – Buchu Compound Tablets | aids normal urinary flow | dandelion, buchu, bearberry, clivers |
| – Waterlex Tablets | to assist normal urinary flow | dandelion, horsetail, bearberry |

| Products | Uses | Ingredients |
|---|---|---|
| – Water Relief Tablets | for relief of premenstrual water retention | bladderwrack, ground ivy, clivers, burdock |
| Heath and Heather Water Relief Tablets | for relief of premenstrual water retention | bladderwrack, ground ivy, clivers, burdock |
| HRI Water Balance | for before or during menstruation and while slimming | buchu, parsley piert, bearberry, dandelion |
| Lane's Cascade Tablets | for elimination of excess water | bearberry, clivers, burdock |
| Modern Herbals Water Retention Tablets | for elimination of excess water | bearberry, clivers, burdock |
| Potter's | | |
| – Antitis | urinary or bladder discomfort, cystitis | buchu, clivers, horsetail, shepherd's purse, bearberry |
| – Diuretabs | for water imbalance | buchu, parsley piert, bearberry, juniper |
| – Kas-Bah Remedy | for urinary and bladder disorders and associated backache | buchu, clivers, horsetail, senna, couchgrass, bearberry |
| – Watershed Mixture | to assist in elimination of excess fluid | wild carrot, pellitory, buchu, juniper, clivers |
| – Watershed Tablets | for water imbalance | buchu, parsley piert, bearberry, juniper |
| Sabalin | for male urinary discomfort | saw palmetto |
| Uvacin | for female bladder discomfort | dandelion, bearberry, peppermint |

## Homoeopathic

| | | |
|---|---|---|
| apis mel | for cystitis with stinging, burning pain | honey-bee |
| belladonna | for cystitis with temperature, headache | deadly nightshade |

| Products | Uses | Ingredients |
|---|---|---|
| **Allopathic** | | |
| Potassium Citrate Mixture BP | for symptomatic relief of cystitis | potassium citrate, citric acid |
| Canesten Oasis | for symptomatic relief of cystitis in women | citric acid, sodium bicarbonate, sodium citrate and carbonate |
| Cymalon | for symptomatic relief of cystitis in women | citric acid, sodium bicarbonate, sodium carbonate |
| Cystemme | for cystitis | sodium citrate and bicarbonate |
| Cystocalm | for symptomatic relief of cystitis in women | sodium citrate |
| Cystofem | for symptomatic relief of cystitis in women | sodium citrate |
| Cystoleve | for symptomatic relief of cystitis in women | sodium citrate |
| Cystopurin | for cystitis | potassium citrate |
| Effercitrate | for cystitis | citric acid, potassium citrate |

# Vitamins, Minerals and Tonics

Vitamins and minerals are essential for health and normal development; they are obtained from the diet. A balanced diet will provide all the vitamins and minerals the body requires for the normal, healthy person. However, some groups of people may need supplements: the elderly, due to poor appetite, poor diet, or disorders affecting their absorption of vitamins and minerals; dieters who may not be eating a balanced diet; vegetarians need vitamin B12 because they don't eat red meat; Asian immigrants may need vitamin D supplements; and alcoholics, due to liver damage, may need vitamin B1, B12 and folic acid. Pregnant and breast-feeding women have additional needs, but pregnant women, and those likely to become pregnant, should not take supplements containing vitamin A without advice from their doctor or antenatal clinic, as excess may cause birth deformities. Diabetics should not take supplements containing chromium as it may enhance insulin sensitivity and so affect blood glucose levels.

Also note that some tonics contain alcohol, which may interact with other medication or affect the ability to drive or operate machinery.

| Product | Uses | Ingredients |
| --- | --- | --- |
| **Herbal** | | |
| Dorwest Damiana and Kola Tablets | for lack of vigour or energy | kola, damiana, saw palmetto |
| Herbal Concepts | | |
| – Daily Tension and Strain Relief | relieves everyday tension and strain | asafetida, valerian, oats, passion-flower |
| – Daily Fatigue Relief | for the alleviation of temporary fatigue and tiredness | kola, damiana, saw palmetto |
| – Daily Overwork and Mental Fatigue Relief | gentle aid to combat the effects of overwork | oats, prickly ash |
| Potter's Chlorophyll Tablets | for relief of temporary tiredness | kola, chlorophyll |
| – Echinacea Elixir | immunostimulant, catarrh, skin conditions | echinacea, wild indigo, fumitory |
| – Elixir Damiana and Saw Palmetto | a restorative, especially for older men | corn silk, damiana, saw palmetto |

| Products | Uses | Ingredients |
|---|---|---|
| – Malted Kelp | mineral source, aid to convalescence | kelp, malt |
| – Strength | for recovery after illness | kola, damiana, saw palmetto |
| Yariba | a pick-me-up for temporary tiredness | kola |

## Homoeopathic

| calc phos | for anaemia during growth spurt, irritability, poor digestion | calcium phosphate |
|---|---|---|
| china | for anaemia due to loss of blood, oversensitivity, chilliness, exhaustion | cinchona |
| ferrum met | for anaemia, with pale face that flushes easily | iron metal |
| nat mur | for anaemia with constipation, headache, and tendency to cold sores | sodium chloride |

## Anthroposophical

Weleda
| – Apatite 6x Comp. Tablets | to aid calcium absorption | apatite, pumpkin |
|---|---|---|
| – Birch Elixir | a spring and autumn tonic | birch, lemon |
| – Blackthorn Elixir | to help in convalescence | blackthorn, lemon |
| – Conchae 5% Comp. Tablets | to aid calcium absorption | conchae, oak |
| – Ferrum Sidereum 6x Tablets | convalescence after colds and flu' | meteoric iron |
| – Fragaria/Urtica Drops | to stimulate the utilisation of iron | wild strawberry, nettle |

## Allopathic

| Calcium and Ergocalciferol Tablets BP | calcium and vitamin supplement | calcium lactate, calcium phosphate, ergocalciferol |
|---|---|---|
| Abidec Drops | vitamin supplement | vitamins A, B1, B2, nicotin-amide, B6, C and D2 |
| Adcal | calcium supplement | calcium carbonate |

| Products | Uses | Ingredients |
|---|---|---|
| Adcal-D3 | calcium and vitamin D supplement | calcium carbonate, cholecalciferol |
| Becosym Forte Tablets | vitamin B supplement | thiamine, vitamin B2, B6, nicotinamide |
| Benerva Tablets | vitamin supplement | thiamine |
| Cacit | calcium supplement | calcium carbonate |
| Cacit D3 | calcium and vitamin D supplement | calcium carbonate, vitamin D3 |
| Calceos | calcium and vitamin D supplement | calcium carbonate, vitamin D3 |
| Calcichew | calcium supplement | calcium carbonate |
| Concavit Capsules Drops and Syrup | vitamin supplement | vitamins A, B1, B2, B6, C, D, E, nicotinamide, calcium, pantothenate |
| Cytacon | vitamin B12 supplement | cyanocobalamin |
| Dalivit | vitamin supplement | vitamins A, B1, B2, B6, C, D2, nicotinamide |
| Effico Tonic | a pick-me-up and appetite promoter | thiamine, nicotinamide, caffeine, gentian compound |
| Ephynal | vitamin E supplement | vitamin E |
| Folicare | folic acid supplement | folic acid |
| Forceval Capsules and Junior Capsules and Powder | to prevent and correct vitamin and mineral-deficiency states | vitamins A, B1, B2, B6, B12, C, D2, E, biotin, nicotinamide, pantothenic acid, folic acid, plus 12 minerals and trace elements |
| Haliborange Infant Drops | vitamin supplement | vitamins A, C and D |
| Labiton | tonic | thiamine, p-aminobenzoic acid, kola, alcohol, caffeine |
| Malt Extract + Cod-Liver Oil | vitamin supplement | malt extract, cod-liver oil, vitamin D |

| Products | Uses | Ingredients |
| --- | --- | --- |
| Metatone | for use in convalescence and debilitating illnesses | thiamine, glycerophosphates of calcium, sodium, manganese |
| Minadex | tonic | vitamins A and D, iron, potassium, calcium, manganese, copper |
| – Multivitamin Syrup | vitamin supplement | vitamins A, B1, B2, B6, C, D, E, nicotinamide |
| Minalka | mineral supplement for relief of muscular pains and joint stiffness | salts of calcium, potassium, sodium, magnesium, cobalt, manganese, copper, zinc, iodine, cholecalciferol |
| Orovite Tablets | for replacement of vitamins lost during illness; for convalescence | vitamins B1, B2, B6, C, nicotinamide |
| Pep | to relieve temporary tiredness | caffeine, dextrose |
| Pharmaton Capsules | for states of exhaustion caused by stress, tiredness, feeling of weakness, lack of vitality, prevention and treatment of symptoms caused by ill-balanced diet or deficient nutrition | ginseng, vitamins A, B1, B2, B6, B12, C, D3, E, nicotinamide, calcium, lecithin, biotin, folic acid, copper, selenium, manganese, magnesium, iron, zinc |
| Preconceive | for prevention of neural tube defects in women planning pregnancy | folic acid |
| Sandocal 400 and 1000 | calcium supplement | calcium salts |
| Seven Seas Vitamin and Mineral Tonic | tonic | vitamins A and D, iron, calcium, potassium, manganese, copper |
| Solvazinc | zinc supplement | zinc sulphate |
| Yeast Vite | for relief of fatigue and tiredness | caffeine, nicotinamide, vitamins B1 and B2 |

# Addenda for Women Only

These products are also listed in the previous specific sections.

| Product | Uses | Ingredients |
|---|---|---|
| **Herbal** | | |
| Gerard House<br>– Water Relief Tablets | for relief of premenstrual water retention | bladderwrack, ground ivy, clivers, burdock |
| Heath and Heather<br>– Raspberry Leaf Tablets | for pain in childbirth | raspberry leaf |
| – Water Relief Tablets | for relief of premenstrual water retention | bladderwrack, ground ivy, clivers, burdock |
| Herbal Concepts<br>– Daily Menopause Relief | for minor conditions associated with the menopause | lime, motherwort, pasque flower, valerian |
| – Period Pain Relief | for premenstrual tension and period pain | lady's-mantle, motherwort, valerian, pasque flower, vervain, false unicorn |
| HRI Water Balance | for before or during menstruation and while slimming | buchu, parsley piert, bearberry, dandelion |
| Lane's<br>– Cascade Tablets | for elimination of excess water | bearberry, clivers, burdock |
| – Athera Tablets | for menopausal symptoms | vervain, senna, clivers, parsley |
| Modern Herbals<br>– Water Retention Tablets | for elimination of excess water | bearberry, clivers, burdock |
| – Menopause Tablets | for relief of minor conditions associated with the menopause | vervain, senna, clivers, parsley |
| Potter's<br>– Black Haw and Golden Seal Elixir | for relief of discomfort in middle-of-life women | black haw, golden seal |
| – Prementaid | for mood-swing aggravation before periods | motherwort, pasque flower, bearberry, valerian |
| – Raspberry Leaf | for menstrual pain | raspberry |

| Products | Uses | Ingredients |
|---|---|---|
| – Wellwoman | for the wellbeing of middle-aged (menopausal) women | yarrow, motherwort, lime flowers, scullcap, valerian |
| Uvacin | for female bladder discomfort | dandelion, bearberry, peppermint |

## Homoeopathic

| | | |
|---|---|---|
| actaea rac | for period pain, irregular, painful, heavy | black cohosh |
| apis mel | for fluid retention, swollen breasts, cystitis | honey-bee |
| belladonna | for cramp-like period pains and cystitis | deadly nightshade |
| bryonia | for menopause with dry vagina and constipation | white bryony |
| calc carb | for PMT and periods with swollen, painful breasts | calcium carbonate |
| calc phos | for heavy painful periods with backache | calcium phosphate |
| graphites | for hot flushes and scanty periods in menopause | graphite |
| ignatia | for periods stopped due to bereavement | st ignatius's bean |
| ipecac | for early period with sickness before and during | ipecacuanha |
| lycopodium | for premenstrual tension and period with headache | club moss |
| nat mur | for PMT and scanty periods with head and backache | sodium chloride |
| pulsatilla | for irregular scanty periods, menopausal hot flushes | pasque flower |
| sepia | for PMT, period and menopausal problems | cuttlefish |
| New Era Tissue Salts: – Combination N | for menstrual pain | calcium phosphate, potassium chloride, potassium phosphate, magnesium phosphate |

| Products | Uses | Ingredients |
|---|---|---|

## Anthroposophical

Wala Pillules
– Melissa/Sepia Comp.

|  | for mild menopausal complaints, including hot flushes, irritability and exhaustion | lemon balm, sepia |
|---|---|---|
| Weleda Menodoron Drops | for relief of menstrual cycle irregularities particularly in young and menopausal women | shepherd's purse, yarrow, oak, nettle, marjoram |

## Allopathic

| Canesten Oasis | for symptomatic relief of cystitis in women | citric acid, sodium bicarbonate, sodium citrate and carbonate |
|---|---|---|
| Cymalon | for symptomatic relief of cystitis in women | citric acid, sodium bicarbonate, sodium carbonate |
| Cystocalm | for symptomatic relief of cystitis in women | sodium citrate |
| Cystofem | for symptomatic relief of cystitis in women | sodium citrate |
| Cystoleve | for symptomatic relief of cystitis in women | sodium citrate |

# Addenda for Men Only

These products are also listed in the previous specific sections.

Problems with urination are common in older men and are frequently due to an enlarged prostate gland (benign prostatic hypertrophy). The cause is unknown, but can be easily treated – see your doctor. The products listed below will help, but medical treatment is required to solve the problem.

| Product | Uses | Ingredients |
|---|---|---|
| **Herbal** | | |
| Potter's Elixir Damiana and Saw Palmetto | restorative, especially for older men | corn silk, damiana, saw palmetto |
| Sabalin | for male urinary discomfort | saw palmetto |

# Part 3

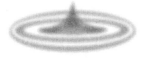

# Glossary

**ABSORBENT** – able to absorb or take up.

**ADJUNCT, ADJUVANT** – an addition to the main therapy.

**ADSORBENT** – able to accumulate on its surface.

**ALCOHOL** – the alcohol we drink in wine is ethanol, this is one of a whole family of chemically related compounds which occur in plants in the form of sterols.

**ALTERNATIVE** – a blood cleanser which detoxifies and promotes restoration of the normal function of an organ or system.

**AMINO ACID** – the basic structural units of protein. There are 22 amino acids that occur naturally; in humans, eight of these are essential amino acids, that is, we must obtain them from our diet, as we are unable to synthesise them ourselves.

**ALKALOID** – a nitrogenous organic base (amine), found in plants, which has a specific physiological action, chiefly on blood vessels and nerves. All taste very bitter, some are toxic; and most are insoluble in water but are soluble in alcohol. As they are alkaline they react with acids to form salts.

**ANALGESIC** – relieves pain.

**ANODYNE** – soothes pain.

**ANTHELMINTIC** – destroying or expelling worms, for example, from the gut.

**ANTHROQUINONE** – substances produced in certain plants which are chemically changed by bacteria in the gut to have a laxative effect, for example, senna.

**ANTI** – means against, having the opposite effect, relieving or reducing an action.

**ANTI-ASTHMATIC** – preventing asthma.

**ANTIBACTERIAL** – inhibiting the growth of bacteria.

**ANTIBILIOUS** – acting on the liver and gall bladder to reduce inflammation and promote bile flow.

**ANTIBIOTIC** – inhibiting the growth of bacteria, or destroying them.

**ANTIFUNGAL** – inhibiting the growth of fungae, or destroying them.

**ANTIHISTAMINE** – prevents the action of histamine (which is released in allergic reactions).

**ANTI-INFECTIVE** – prevents infection by stimulating the immune system.

**ANTI-INFLAMMATORY** – reducing inflammation.

**ANTIMICROBIAL** – destroying or inhibiting the growth of micro-organisms, bacteria, fungae, viruses.

**ANTIOXIDANT** – a group of vitamins (A, C and E) and the mineral (selenium) which protect against free radicals.

**ANTIPRURITIC** – reducing itchiness.

**ANTIPYRETIC** – reducing the body temperature, as in fever, i.e. a **FEBRIFUGE**.

**ANTIRHEUMATIC** – relieving rheumatism and arthritis.

**ANTISCORBUTIC** – a substance that prevents scurvy, for example, vitamin C.

**ANTISEPTIC** – used to cleanse wounds and prevent infection, **ANTIMICROBIAL**.

**ANTISPASMODIC** – relieving spasm by relaxing the muscle.

**ANTITUSSIVE** – reducing the severity of coughs and easing expectoration.

**ANTIVIRAL** – inhibiting the growth of viruses.

**APERIENT** – a medicine that produces a normal bowel movement.

**APHRODISIAC** – a substance that excites sexual desire.

**APNOEA** – cessation of breathing, can be temporary or for a prolonged period.

**AROMATIC**- having an aroma.

**ARTERIOSCLEROSIS** – hardening of the arteries
– see **ATHEROSCLEROSIS**.

**ASTRINGENT** – having the power to contract organic tissue, such as blood vessels, mucous membranes etc., which has the effect of reducing secretion or excretion. The tannin content of a herb is responsible for this action.

**ATHEROSCLEROSIS** – the thickening of the inner wall of arteries by deposition of cholesterol and other substances – this is the most significant form of arteriosclerosis.

**ATOPIC** – allergic response or hypersensitivity of an inherited nature, but not to a specific substance.

**BACTERICIDAL** – destroys bacteria.

**BENIGN** – harmless.

**BITTER** – stimulates the digestion and hence improves appetite.

**CARDIAC** – pertaining to the heart.

**CARMINATIVE** – the effect of expelling flatulence or wind from the stomach and intestines. Many essential oils contained in herbs are carminative; they act by toning the mucous surfaces of the intestines and increasing peristaltic action.

**CATARRH** – increased mucous production associated with inflammation of mucous membranes.

**CHOLAGOGUE** – acting to increase the secretion of bile and its expulsion from the gall bladder.

**CONTACT DERMATITIS** – an allergic response, usually an itchy rash, in response to contact with a substance, for example, detergents, plants, nickel, cosmetics.

**COUMARIN** – they are anticoagulant substances found in plants and trees – they prevent blood from clotting.

**COUNTERIRRITANT** – when applied to the skin, it causes a superficial irritation which increases blood flow to the area, so speeding up the removal of toxins and hence relieving the inflammation of the deeper tissues.

**DECONGESTANT** – relieves congestion, especially of the nose.

**DEMULCENT** – soothing, offering protection and relief to inflamed or irritated mucous membranes.

**DIAPHORETIC** – promoting perspiration, a process of internal cleansing.

**DILUENT**- used to dilute or weaken the strength of something.

**DIURETIC** – a substance that stimulates the kidneys to increase urine production.

**DYSPEPSIA** – indigestion.

**ECZEMA** – inflammation of the skin, usually with itching and sometimes with scaling and blisters, sometimes caused by an allergy but often of no known cause.

**EMETIC** – causes vomiting.

**EMMENAGOGUE** – a substance which induces menstruation, a uterine tonic and stimulant.

**EMOLLIENT** – soothes and softens the skin.

**EMULSIFIER** – a substance , for example, acacia*, that is used to assist in making an emulsion, which is a mixture of oil and water.

**EXCIPIENT** – an inactive ingredient incorporated into a medicine to maintain its consistency, for example, emulsifiers in creams and lotions, binders in tablets.

**EXPECTORANT** – promoting the liquefaction and expulsion of mucous from the body, particularly the respiratory tract.

**FEBRIFUGE** – reduces fever.

**FIXED OIL** – on heating, fixed oils do not volatilise, as essential oils do, but will eventually decompose if too much heat is applied. They are used for cooking, for example, olive oil*.

**FLATULENCE** – abdominal discomfort due to gas, relieved by belching or passage of wind.

**FLAVONOID** – also called flavones, they are naturally occurring chemicals which prevent the deposit of fatty materials in the blood vessels. Their main actions are diuretic, antispasmodic and antiseptic; they lower blood pressure, add tone to relaxed blood vessels and strengthen fragile capillaries. They are also the pigments responsible for the colour of flowers and fruits.

**FREE RADICALS** – harmful and aggressive molecules which attack cells in our body, causing them to deteriorate. They are neutralised by **ANTIOXIDANTS**.

**GALACTOGOGUE** – stimulating production of breast milk and increasing the flow.

**GLYCERIDES** – esters produced by action of an acid on an alcohol such as glycerol.

**GLYCOSIDES** – an organic substance which is made up of a sugar (glycone) and a non-sugar (aglycone). The two parts can be separated by heating in dilute acid or by use of an enzyme. The cardiac glycosides, found in foxglove* are the best known. The flavonoid glycosides are another important group, found particularly in the Labiatae family of plants (lavender*, rosemary*, sage, thyme* etc).

**HAEMORRHOIDS** – swollen or varicose veins in the lining of the anus.

**HAEMOSTATIC** – stops bleeding.

**HEPATIC** – pertaining to the liver.

**HYPERLIPIDAEMIA** – high cholesterol level.

**HYPERPLASIA** – an overgrowth due to an excessive multiplication of cells.

**HYPERTENSION** – high blood pressure.

**HYPOTENSION** – low blood pressure.

**ICHTHYOSIS** – a rare, inherited skin condition due to an abnormality in keratin production.

**IMPETIGO** – a highly contagious bacterial skin infection, usually around the nose and mouth – treatment is with antibiotic cream or ointment.

**INERT** – inactive.

**INSECTICIDE** – a substance that kills insects.

**IRIDOID** – a type of organic molecule found in plants and animals, for example, terpenes.

**ISOMER** – having the same molecular formula but shaped differently, for example, a mirror image.

**KERATOLYTIC** – loosening and removing the tough outer layers of the skin.

**LATEX** – the milky juice of some plants.

**LAXATIVE** – encourages bowel movements.

**MALIGNANT** – harmful, likely to cause death.

**METABOLISM** – a collective term for all the chemical processes that take place in the body. Catabolism is a breaking down (for example, of glucose to produce energy), whilst anabolism is a building up (for example, of proteins from amino acids). The metabolic rate is controlled by various hormones, for example, adrenalin, insulin and thyroid hormones.

**MORBIDITY** – incidence of illness.

**MUCILAGE** – a sticky mixture of carbohydrates found in plants, which may be of value for inflamed surfaces due to their healing properties.

Also a term used pharmaceutically for a viscous mixture prepared from, for example, acacia* or tragacanth*, and liquid.

**NARCOTIC** – a drug which causes stupor and relieves pain.

**NB** – Nota bene – Latin for note well.

**NERVINE** – restoring the nerves, mildly tranquillising.

**NUTRIENT** – provides nourishment as a food.

**OSMOTIC** – causing diffusion of liquids through a semi-permeable membrane.

**PARASITICIDE** – kills parasites.

**PECTORAL** – having an effect on the lungs.

**PERINEAL** – refers to the part of the body between the genitals and the anus.

**PERIPHERAL** – near the surface of the body.

**PERISTALSIS** – waves of contraction in the alimentary canal, which force the contents along.

**PHENOLS** and **PHENOLIC ACIDS** – a class of aromatic compounds which are weak acids but which react as alcohols.

**PHOTOSENSITIVITY** – an abnormal reaction to sunlight, usually a rash, caused by certain drugs, dyes, chemicals and certain plants, for example, mustard.

**PHYTOSTEROL** – a substance , similar to cholesterol, found in plants.

**POSTPARTUM** – after giving birth.

**PROSTAGLANDIN** – a number of fatty acids made by the body that act in a similar way to hormones. First found in semen, they are named after the prostate gland, but we now know they are produced throughout the body and have a range of effects, including causing the pain and inflammation of damaged tissue, protecting the lining of the stomach and duodenum against ulceration, and stimulating contractions during labour.

**PROSTATIC** – of the prostate gland.

**PSORIASIS** – a skin disease characterised by thickened patches of inflamed, red skin.

**PURGATIVE** – has a more drastic action than a laxative, usually given with a carminative to prevent griping.

**QUINONE** – a type of organic compound found in plants.

**REFRIGERANT** – relieving thirst and giving a feeling of coolness.

**RESIN** – a solid or semi-solid substance produced by certain plants and trees. They may be produced in association with gum or oil. They are insoluble in water but soluble in alcohol.

**RUBEFACIENT** – causing the skin to redden, so increasing blood flow and removal of toxins.

**SAPONIN** – they are glycosides which produce a soap-like foaming effect in water. They have a detergent action on mucous membranes.

**SEDATIVE** – reduces stress and anxiety.

**SENSITIVITY** – a heightened response to something.

**SPASMOLYTIC** – antispasmodic.

**STEROL** – a waxy, steroid alcohol, such as cholesterol.

**STIMULANT** – increases physiological activity, for example, the circulation, the nervous system, prostaglandin synthesis. Different herbs stimulate different parts of the body.

**STOMACHIC** – used to treat stomach disorders.

**TANNIN** – they are water soluble, phenolic compounds which have a constricting effect. They are acid astringents that coagulate proteins and inhibit the deposition of fatty deposits in the body.

**TERPENE** – a type of hydrocarbon found in plants and trees, for example, turpentine*.

**THIXOTROPIC** – something that exhibits a change in viscosity when shaken or stirred, for example, non-drip paint.

**TONIC** – improves the sense of wellbeing by improving physiological functioning of the body.

**TOPICAL** – applied to the surface of the body.

**TOXIC** – harmful or poisonous.

**URTICARIA** – a skin condition with raised wheals and inflammation, as in nettle rash.

**UTERINE** – of the womb.

**WART** – a common, contagious but harmless growth on skin or mucous membranes, caused by a viral infection. They can appear anywhere on the body – hands, feet, face, knees, genitals.

**VERRUCA** – a wart on the sole of the foot, otherwise known as a plantar wart – they are flattened simply because of the pressure applied to them by standing.

**VULNERARY** – good for healing wounds.

# List of Herbs by their Actions

## ALTERNATIVES
Alfalfa, Bladderwrack, Blue Flag, Burdock, Celandine, Clivers, Clover, Dandelion, Devil's Claw, Dock, Echinacea, Elder, Fringe Tree, Garlic, Ginseng, Goldenseal, Marigold, Meadowsweet, Nettle, Pasque Flower, Poke Root, Polypody, Sarsaparilla, Wild Indigo.

## ANALGESICS or ANODYNES
Aconite, Aloe Vera, Angelica, Birch, Black Cohosh, Boneset, Camphor, Chamomile, Clove, Devil's Claw, Feverfew, Gelsemium, Gentian, Henbane, Hops, Jamaica Dogwood, Kava, Lignum Vitae, Linseed, Lobelia, Maté, Meadow Saffron, Mistletoe, Opium Poppy, Pasque Flower, Passion Flower, Poke Root, Poplar, Prickly Ash, Rosemary, Scullcap, Skunk Cabbage, St John's Wort, Thornapple, Valerian, Vervain, Wild Lettuce, Wild Yam, Willow, Wintergreen.

## ANTHELMINTICS
Asafetida, Betel, Bryony (White), Butternut, Castor, Garlic, Gentian, Hyssop, Male Fern, Neem, Pumpkin, Rue, Savin, Senna, Thyme.

## ANTI-ANAEMICS
Alfalfa, Bladderwrack, Burdock, Couch Grass, Devil's Claw, Meadowsweet, Nettle, Parsley, Wild Strawberry.

## ANTI-ASTHMATICS
Black Haw, Comfrey, Elecampne, Ephedra, Gelsemium, Irish Moss, Lobelia, Onion, Storax, Sundew, Thornapple, Wild Strawberry, Wild Yam.

## ANTIBILIOUS
Barberry, Black Root, Centaury, Chamomile, Dandelion, Dock, Fringe Tree, Fumitory, Goldenseal, Holy Thistle, Hops, Turmeric, Vervain, Wahoo, Wild Yam.

## ANTIBIOTICS

Aloe Vera, Blue Flag, Buchu, Burdock, Capsicum, Clove, Clover, Echinacea, Garlic, Goldenseal, Holy Thistle, Horseradish, Iceland Moss, Juniper, Lobelia, Lungwort, Mustard, Onion, Poke Root, Propolis, Royal Jelly, Thyme, Wild Indigo.

## ANTICATARRHALS

Angelica, Bayberry, Benzoin, Capsicum, Coltsfoot, Comfrey, Elder, Elecampne, Eyebright, Fenugreek, Garlic, Ginger, Goldenseal, Horehound, Hyssop, Iceland Moss, Irish Moss, Ivy (Ground), Juniper, Liquorice, Lovage, Marshmallow, Matricaria, Myrrh, Parsley, Poke Root, Skunk Cabbage, Wild Indigo, Yarrow.

## ANTICHOLESTEROLS

Alfalfa, Artichoke, Barley, Corn, Garlic, Ginger, Ginseng, Milk Thistle, Red Vine, Sunflower.

## ANTICOAGULANTS

Alfalfa, Bayberry, Garlic, Ginseng, Lime.

## ANTIDEPRESSANTS

Celery, Chamomile, Damiana, Gingko, Kola, Lavender, Lemon Balm, Mistletoe, Oats, Rosemary, Scullcap, St John's Wort, Valerian, Vervain.

## ANTIDIARRHOEALS

Arrowroot, Cinnamon, Hemlock Spruce, Holy Thistle, Ispahula, Kola, Nutmeg, Oak, Opium Poppy, Rhatany.

## ANTI-EMETICS

Barberry, Capsicum, Cinnamon, Clove, Coffee, Dill, Elecampne, Fennel, Fringe Tree, Gentian, Ginger, Iceland Moss, Lavender, Marigold, Meadowsweet, Nutmeg, Peppermint.

## ANTIFUNGALS

Aloe Vera, Aniseed, Bay, Bittersweet, Burdock, Calumba, Castor, Celandine, Echinacea, Eucalyptus, Garlic, Gingko, Ivy (Ground), Marigold, Myrrh, Poke Root, Propolis, Tea Tree, Thyme, Wild Indigo, Witch Hazel.

## ANTIGOUTS

Black Cohosh, Boldo, Burdock, Celery, Couch Grass, Dandelion, Devil's Claw, Gravel Root, Horseradish, Meadowsweet, Sarsaparilla, Valerian, Wild Lettuce, Willow, Yarrow.

## ANTIHISTAMINES

Burdock, Butterbur, Clove, Echinacea, Elder, Ephedra, Eyebright, Garlic, Goldenseal, Lobelia, Marigold, Marshmallow, Parsley, Peppermint, Sage.

## ANTI-INFECTIVES – see IMMUNE STIMULANTS

## ANTI-INFLAMMATORIES

Asafetida, Barberry, Birch, Black Cohosh, Black Haw, Blackthorn, Blue Flag, Boldo, Buckbean, Burdock, Butterbur, Cat's Claw, Celery, Chamomile, Clivers, Clover, Comfrey, Devil's Claw, Dock, Elder, Eyebright, Fennel, Feverfew, Fumitory, Gentian, Ginger, Ginseng, Horehound, Horse Chestnut, Ipecacuahna, Jamaica Dogwood, Juniper, Lemon, Lignum Vitae, Liquorice, Marigold, Marshmallow, Matricaria, Meadow Saffron, Meadowsweet, Mistletoe, Myrrh, Nutmeg, Oak, Parsley, Pellitory, Pineapple, Poke Root, Poplar, Primula, Propolis, Red Vine, Rhubarb, Rosemary, Rue, Safflower, Snake Root, Stone Root, St John's Wort, Turmeric, Vervain, Wild Pansy, Wild Yam, Willow, Wintergreen, Witch Hazel.

## ANTIMICROBIALS

Aloe Vera, Angelica, Aniseed, Barberry, Bayberry, Bearberry, Benzoin, Buchu, Camphor, Caraway, Catechu, Capsicum, Celandine, Cinnamon, Clove, Corn Silk, Coriander, Echinacea, Elecampne, Eucalyptus, Fennel, Garlic, Gentian, Gingko, Goldenseal, Hemlock Spruce, Hops, Juniper, Kava, Lavender, Lemon Balm, Lignum Vitae, Liquorice, Lovage, Marigold, Marjoram, Marshmallow, Matricaria, Meadowsweet, Myrrh, Olive, Parsley, Pasque Flower, Peppermint, Peru Balsam, Propolis, Rosemary, Rue, Sage, St John's Wort, Tea Tree, Thyme, Turmeric, Wild Indigo, Yarrow.

## ANTI-OBESITY

Black Cohosh, Bladderwrack, Blue Flag, Boldo, Chickweed, Clivers, Dandelion, Fennel, Garlic, Maté, Motherwort, Parsley.

## ANTIOXIDANTS

Alfalfa, Artichoke, Bilberry, Comfrey, Garlic, Ginseng, Goldenseal, Irish Moss, Jojoba, Parsley, Turmeric, Watercress.

## ANTIPRURITIC

Boneset, Cade, Chickweed, Clover, Dandelion, Devil's Claw, Echinacea, Marigold, Nettle, Peppermint, Poke Root, Sarsaparilla, Wild Yam, Witch Hazel.

## ANTIRHEUMATICS

Barberry, Black Cohosh, Bladderwrack, Blue Flag, Bittersweet, Boneset, Buckbean, Burdock, Capsicum, Celery, Chickweed, Couch Grass, Dandelion, Devil's Claw, Dock, Elder, Gravel Root, Juniper, Lavender, Lignum Vitae, Meadowsweet, Nettle, Parsley, Poke Root, Poplar, Prickly Ash, Sarsaparilla, Wild Yam, Willow, Wintergreen, Yarrow.

## ANTISCORBUTICS

Blue Flag, Buckbean, Burdock, Chickweed, Clivers, Dock, Lemon, Nettle, Orange, Sarsaparilla, Scurvy Grass, Shepherd's Purse, Watercress.

## ANTISEPTICS

Barberry, Bay, Bearberry, Benzoin, Bergamot, Black Root, Boldo, Buchu, Cade, Cajuput, Camphor, Catechu, Celery, Cinchona, Cinnamon, Cranberry, Echinacea, Elder, Elecampne, Eucalyptus, Garlic, Gentian, Goldenseal, Hemlock Spruce, Horehound, Horseradish, Hydrangea, Juniper, Lavender, Marigold, Matricaria, Myrrh, Nettle, Oak, Olive, Onion, Peppermint, Poke Root, Poplar, Pumilio Pine, Rhubarb, Rosemary, Sage, Sarsaparilla, Saw Palmetto, Shepherd's Purse, Spurge, Storax, Tea Tree, Thyme, Tolu, Wild Indigo, Willow, Wintergreen.

## ANTISPASMODICS

Angelica, Aniseed, Asafetida, Belladonna, Bergamot, Black Cohosh, Black Haw, Butterbur, Cajuput, Camphor, Capsicum, Caraway, Cardamom, Celandine, Chamomile, Clove, Clover, Devil's Claw, Dill, Elecampne, Ephedra, Eucalyptus, Fennel, Fumitory, Gelsemium, Ginger, Hawthorn, Henbane, Hops, Horehound, Hyssop, Ipecacuahna, Jamaica Dogwood, Kava, Lavender, Lemon Balm, Lime, Liquorice, Lobelia, Lovage, Marjoram, Matricaria, Mistletoe, Motherwort, Nutmeg, Oats, Onion, Opium Poppy, Parsley, Pasque Flower, Passion Flower, Peony, Peppermint, Pleurisy Root, Prickly Ash, Primula, Raspberry, Rosemary, Rue, Sage, Saw Palmetto, Scullcap, Skunk Cabbage, Spearmint, Spurge, Squill, Sundew, Sweet Flag, Thornapple, Thyme, Valerian, Vervain, Wild Carrot, Wild Lettuce, Wild Strawberry, Wild Yam, Yarrow.

## ANTITUSSIVES

Angelica, Coltsfoot, Comfrey, Elecampne, Fenugreek, Garlic, Horehound, Hyssop, Iceland Moss, Irish Moss, Jamaica Dogwood, Linseed, Liquorice, Lobelia, Marshmallow, Opium Poppy, Pleurisy Root, Poplar, Slippery Elm, Squill, Sundew, Thyme, Wild Lettuce.

## ANTIVIRALS

Aloe Vera, Boneset, Burdock, Echinacea, Elder, Elecampne, Eucalyptus, Garlic, Goldenseal, Lemon Balm, Liquorice, Mandrake, Marjoram, Pasque Flower, Savin, Wild Indigo, Yarrow.

## APERIENTS – see LAXATIVES

## APHRODISIACS

Angelica, Arnica, Burdock, Celery, Damiana, Ginseng, Guarana, Honey, Kola, Royal Jelly, Saw Palmetto.

## AROMATICS

Allspice, Angelica, Aniseed, Bergamot, Camphor, Caraway, Cardamom, Celery, Centaury, Cinnamon, Clove, Coriander, Dill, Eucalyptus, Fennel, Ginger, Hops, Hyssop, Ivy (Ground), Juniper, Lavender, Lemon, Lemon Balm, Lovage, Meadowsweet, Orange, Parsley, Peppermint, Pine, Rosemary, Sage, Spearmint, St John's Wort, Valerian, Vervain.

## ASTRINGENTS

Agrimony, Aloe Vera, Bayberry, Bearberry, Benzoin, Betel, Bilberry, Birch, Black Cohosh, Blackberry, Blackthorn, Blue Flag, Boneset, Catechu, Cinchona, Cinnamon, Clivers, Clover, Comfrey, Devil's Claw, Dock, Elder, Elecampne, Eyebright, Gravel Root, Guarana, Hartstongue, Hawthorn, Hemlock Spruce, Horse Chestnut, Horsetail, Ivy (Ground), Kola, Lime, Loosestrife, Lungwort, Meadowsweet, Myrrh, Nettle, Oak, Olive, Opium Poppy, Parsley Piert, Pilewort, Poison Ivy, Poison Oak, Poplar, Primula, Quince, Raspberry, Red Vine, Rhatany, Rhubarb, Rose, Rosemary, Sage, Shepherd's Purse, Scullcap, Stone Root, St John's Wort, Tea, Vervain, Wild Strawberry, Willow, Wintergreen, Witch Hazel, Yarrow.

## BITTERS

Barberry, Birch, Boneset, Buckbean, Buckthorn, Calumba, Centaury, Cinchona, Devil's Claw, Feverfew, Fumitory, Gentian, Goldenseal, Guarana, Holy Thistle, Hops, Horehound, Ivy (Ground), Juniper, Matricaria, Nux Vomica, Oak, Parsley, Passion Flower, Poplar, Prickly Ash, Rue, Scullcap, Sweet Flag, Vervain, Wild Indigo, Wild Strawberry, Yarrow.

## CARDIACS

Asparagus, Butterbur, Capsicum, Ephedra, Foxglove, Garlic, Hawthorn, Kola, Lime, Mistletoe, Motherwort, Rosemary, St John's Wort, Wahoo, Yarrow.

## CARMINATIVES

Allspice, Angelica, Aniseed, Asafetida, Bay, Benzoin, Bergamot, Cajuput, Calumba, Capsicum, Caraway, Cardamom, Celery, Centaury, Chamomile, Cinnamon, Clove, Coriander, Dill, Fennel, Feverfew, Garlic, Gentian, Ginger, Holy Thistle, Horseradish, Hyssop, Juniper, Kava, Lavender, Lemon Balm, Linseed, Lovage, Mace, Marjoram, Matricaria, Mustard, Nutmeg, Onion, Orange, Parsley, Peppermint, Pleurisy Root, Prickly Ash, Rosemary, Sage, Spearmint, Sweet Flag, Thyme, Valerian, Wild Carrot, Yarrow.

## CHOLAGOGUES

Aloe Vera, Artichoke, Barberry, Belladonna, Black Root, Blue Flag, Boldo, Boneset, Butternut, Celandine, Dandelion, Devil's Claw, Dock, Fringe Tree, Fumitory, Gentian, Goldenseal, Horehound, Liquorice, Turmeric, Wahoo, Wild Yam.

## COUNTERIRRITANTS

Arnica, Belladonna, Cajuput, Camphor, Capsicum, Eucalyptus, Horseradish, Mustard, Turpentine, Wintergreen.

## DECONGESTANTS

Chamomile, Elder, Eucalyptus, Garlic, Goldenseal, Hyssop, Lobelia, Menthol, Myrrh, Peppermint, Poke Root, Pumilio Pine, Thyme, Wild Indigo.

## DEMULCENTS

Almond, Barley, Borage, Chickweed, Coltsfoot, Comfrey, Couch Grass, Fig, Fenugreek, Flax, Iceland Moss, Ispaghula, Linseed, Liquorice, Lungwort, Marshmallow, Meadowsweet, Olive, Parsley Piert, Pellitory, Pilewort, Pumpkin, Quince, Slippery Elm, Sundew, Tragacanth.

## DIAPHORETICS

Aconite, Aloe Vera, Angelica, Bay, Bayberry, Blackcurrant, Black Root, Boneset, Buchu, Burdock, Camphor, Capsicum, Clivers, Elder, Elecampne, Ephedra, Fumitory, Garlic, Gelsemium, Ginger, Hemlock Spruce, Holy Thistle, Horehound, Horseradish, Hyssop, Ipecacuahna, Ivy (Ground), Lime, Lobelia, Lovage, Marigold, Marjoram, Motherwort, Opium Poppy, Pasque Flower, Peppermint, Pleurisy Root, Prickly Ash, Pumilio Pine, Rosemary, Sarsaparilla, Skunk Cabbage, Slippery Elm, Snake Root, Thyme, Vervain, Wild Lettuce, Wild Pansy, Yarrow.

## DIURETICS

Agrimony, Angelica, Arnica, Bay, Bilberry, Birch, Bittersweet, Black Cohosh, Blackcurrant, Blackthorn, Blue Flag, Boldo, Buchu, Buckthorn, Burdock, Butterbur, Carob, Celandine, Celery, Clivers, Clover, Club Moss, Cocoa, Coffee, Couch Grass, Damiana, Dandelion, Elder, Fennel, Foxglove, Fringe Tree, Fumitory, Garlic, Gravel Root, Guarana, Hartstongue, Hawthorn, Henbane, Hops, Horseradish, Horsetail, Hydrangea, Ivy (Ground), Juniper, Kava, Kola, Larch, Lemon, Lignum Vitae, Lime, Lovage, Maté, Meadowsweet, Motherwort, Mustard, Nettle, Nux Vomica, Onion, Parsley, Parsley Piert, Pellitory, Poplar, Pumpkin, Red Vine, Rose, Safflower, Sarsaparilla, Savin, Saw Palmetto, Scurvy Grass, Shepherd's Purse, Skunk Cabbage, Snake Root, Squill, Stone Root, St John's Wort, Sunflower, Tea, Thyme, Vervain, Watercress, Wintergreen, Wild Carrot, Wild Lettuce, Wild Pansy, Wild Strawberry, Wild Yam.

## EMETICS

Black Root, Boneset, Castor, Chamomile, Elder, Holy Thistle, Ipecacuahna, Laurel, Lobelia, Meadow Saffron, Mustard, Nux Vomica, Poke Root, Primula, Sabadilla, Snake Root, Squill, Vervain, Wild Indigo.

## EMMENAGOGUES

Agnus Castus, Aloes, Angelica, Barberry, Barley, Black Cohosh, Black Haw, Celandine, Celery, Chamomile, False Unicorn Root, Feverfew, Goldenseal, Holy Thistle, Lady's Mantle, Marigold, Parsley, Pasque Flower, Peppermint, Poke Root, Raspberry, Red Vine, Rosemary, Safflower, Senna, Shepherd's Purse, St John's Wort, Valerian, Vervain, Yarrow.

## EMOLLIENTS

Almond, Angelica, Arachis, Borage, Castor, Chickweed, Cocoa, Coconut, Comfrey, Elecampne, Fenugreek, Fig, Flax, Irish Moss, Linseed, Liquorice, Lungwort, Marshmallow, Oats, Olive, Rape, Slippery Elm, Soya, Tragacanth.

## EXPECTORANTS

Aniseed, Asafetida, Benzoin, Bittersweet, Black Cohosh, Boneset, Cajuput, Caraway, Cardamom, Chickweed, Clover, Coltsfoot, Comfrey, Elder, Elecampne, Eucalyptus, Fennel, Fenugreek, Flax, Garlic, Ginger, Goldenseal, Holy Thistle, Horehound, Hyssop, Iceland Moss, Irish Moss, Ipecacuahna, Ivy (Ground), Larch, Lignum Vitae, Lime, Linseed, Liquorice, Lobelia, Loosestrife, Lovage, Lungwort, Marshmallow, Myrrh, Nettle, Onion, Opium Poppy, Parsley, Pleurisy Root, Polypody, Poplar, Primula, Pumilio Pine, Saw Palmetto, Skunk Cabbage, Slippery Elm, Snake Root, Spurge, Squill, Storax, St John's Wort, Sundew, Sunflower, Thyme, Tolu, Valerian, Watercress, Wild Pansy, Wild Strawberry, Wintergreen.

## FEBRIFUGES

Aconite, Angelica, Barberry, Bittersweet, Blackcurrant, Boneset, Borage, Buckbean, Calumba, Capsicum, Cinchona, Elder, Eucalyptus, Gelsemium, Gentian, Guarana, Holy Thistle, Horse Chestnut, Hyssop, Lemon Balm, Lobelia, Marigold, Peppermint, Pleurisy Root, Poplar, Prickly Ash, Raspberry, Sage, Thyme, Wild Indigo, Willow, Yarrow.

## GALACTOGOGUES

Agnus Castus, Celery, Fennel, Fenugreek, Holy Thistle, Nettle, Raspberry, Vervain, Wintergreen.

## HAEMOSTATICS

Alginates, Aloe Vera, Bayberry, Bearberry, Blackberry, Capsicum, Cinnamon, Comfrey, Dock, Ephedra, Goldenseal, Holy Thistle, Horsetail, Lady's Mantle, Loosestrife, Marigold, Oak, Red Vine, Rhatany, Shepherd's Purse, St John's Wort, Turmeric, Vervain, Wild Strawberry, Witch Hazel, Yarrow.

## HEALING

Comfrey, Fenugreek, Horsetail, Iceland Moss, Marigold, Marshmallow, Meadowsweet, Witch Hazel.

## HEPATICS

Agrimony, Barberry, Butternut, Black Root, Blue Flag, Boldo, Buckbean, Celandine, Centaury, Clivers, Dandelion, Dock, Fringe Tree, Fumitory, Gentian, Goldenseal, Hyssop, Liquorice, Milk Thistle, Prickly Ash, Stone Root, Turmeric, Wahoo, Wild Indigo, Wild Yam.

## HYPNOTICS

Aniseed, Fennel, Henbane, Hops, Jamaica Dogwood, Mistletoe, Opium Poppy, Passion Flower, Scullcap, Wild Lettuce, Valerian.

## IMMUNE STIMULANTS

Blue Flag, Buchu, Butterbur, Cat's Claw, Clover, Comfrey, Devil's Claw, Echinacea, Elder, Feverfew, Garlic, Goldenseal, Holy Thistle, Horseradish, Juniper, Marigold, Myrrh, Poke Root, Royal Jelly, Sabadilla, Stavesacre, Tea Tree, Thyme, Tragacanth, Watercress, Wild Indigo.

## INSECTICIDES

Arnica, Clove, Comfrey, Eucalyptus, Marigold, Myrrh, Neem, Pyrethrum, Sabadilla, St John's Wort.

## INSECT REPELLENTS

Citronella, Clove, Garlic, Lavender, Lemon Balm, Neem, Peppermint, Thyme.

## LAXATIVES

Agar, Aloes, Almond, Arachis, Barberry, Black Root, Blue Flag, Boldo, Boneset, Bran, Bryony (White), Buckbean, Buckthorn, Burdock, Butternut, Cascara, Castor, Celandine, Chicory, Clivers, Club Moss, Couch Grass, Damiana, Dandelion, Dock, Dog's Mercury, Elder, Fenugreek, Fig, Fringe Tree, Fumitory, Goldenseal, Hartstongue, Honey, Horseradish, Hydrangea, Irish Moss, Ispaghula, Ivy (Ground), Lignum Vitae, Linseed, Liquorice, Meadow Saffron, Motherwort, Olive, Parsley, Pellitory, Pleurisy Root, Poke Root, Rhubarb, Rose, Sabadilla, Safflower, Scurvy Grass, Senna, Stavesacre, Sterculia, Tragacanth, Wahoo, Walnut, Wild Indigo, Wild Pansy, Wild Strawberry.

## NARCOTICS

Belladonna, Bittersweet, Guarana, Henbane, Horse Chestnut, Laurel, Mistletoe, Passion Flower, Poison Ivy, Opium Poppy, Poke Root, Skunk Cabbage, Thornapple, Wild Lettuce.

## NERVINES

Asafetida, Black Cohosh, Black Haw, Celery, Damiana, False Unicorn Root, Guarana, Hops, Kola, Lavender, Lime, Mistletoe, Motherwort, Oats, Pasque Flower, Poke Root, Scullcap, St John's Wort, Valerian, Vervain, Wild Yam.

## NUTRIENTS

Alfalfa, Almonds, Arachis, Arrowroot, Barley, Carob, Cocoa, Coconut, Corn, Fenugreek, Fig, Iceland Moss, Irish Moss, Oats, Olive, Saw Palmetto, Slippery Elm, Soya, Sunflower, Watercress.

## PARASITICIDES

Aniseed, Cinnamon, Garlic, Neem, Peru Balsam, Poke Root, Rosemary, Rue, Stavesacre, Storax, Tolu.

## PURGATIVES – see LAXATIVES

## REFRIGERANTS

Bilberry, Blackcurrant, Borage, Chickweed, Lemon, Lime, Liquorice, Parsley Piert, Pellitory, Raspberry.

## RUBEFACIENTS

Bryony (Black), Cajuput, Camphor, Capsicum, Clove, Garlic, Ginger, Horseradish, Mustard, Pellitory, Peppermint, Poison Ivy, Pumilio Pine, Rue, Thyme, Turpentine, Wintergreen.

## SEDATIVES

Aconite, Angelica, Asafetida, Barberry, Belladonna, Black Cohosh, Boldo, Calumba, Camphor, Chamomile, Clover, Devil's Claw, Evening Primrose, Foxglove, Gelsemium, Henbane, Hops, Horehound, Jamaica Dogwood, Kava, Lavender, Lemon Balm, Lime, Lobelia, Lovage, Matricaria, Mistletoe, Motherwort, Opium Poppy, Pasque Flower, Passion Flower, Poppy, Rosemary, Saw Palmetto, Scullcap, Skunk Cabbage, St John's Wort, Thornapple, Thyme, Valerian, Vervain, Wild Lettuce, Wild Strawberry, Wild Yam.

## STIMULANTS

Allspice, Angelica, Arnica, Barberry, Bayberry, Betel, Bittersweet, Blue Flag, Boneset, Buchu, Butterbur, Calamus, Capsicum, Caraway, Cardamom, Celery, Cinnamon, Clove, Cocoa, Coffee, Coriander, Damiana, Dill, Elder, Elecampne, Ephedra, Eucalyptus, Fennel, Feverfew, Fringe Tree, Garlic, Ginger, Ginseng, Goldenseal, Guarana, Holy Thistle, Horseradish, Ipecacuahna, Ivy (Ground), Juniper, Kava, Kola, Larch, Lavender, Lime, Lobelia, Lovage, Mace, Maté, Marigold, Marjoram, Motherwort, Mustard, Nettle, Nutmeg, Nux Vomica, Oats, Peppermint, Peru Balsam, Poison Ivy, Poplar, Prickly Ash, Raspberry, Rosemary, Rue, Sage, Sarsaparilla, Saw Palmetto, Scurvy Grass, Shepherd's Purse, Spearmint, Squill, Storax, Tea, Tolu, Valerian, Wahoo, Watercress, Wintergreen.

## STOMACHICS

Agrimony, Allspice, Angelica, Artichoke, Bay, Black Root, Calamus, Calumba, Capsicum, Caraway, Cardamom, Cat's Claw, Celery, Centaury, Chamomile, Cinnamon, Comfrey, Coriander, Damiana, Dandelion, Devil's Claw, Dill, Elecampne, Fennel, Fenugreek, Fringe Tree, Gentian, Ginger, Ginseng, Goldenseal, Hops, Iceland Moss, Irish Moss, Juniper, Lady's Mantle, Liquorice, Marigold, Marshmallow, Matricaria, Meadowsweet, Nutmeg, Orange, Parsley, Peppermint, Rhubarb, Slippery Elm, Thyme, Valerian, Wahoo, Wild Carrot, Wild Yam.

## TONICS

Agrimony, Angelica, Barberry, Bayberry, Bergamot, Black Root, Blackberry, Blackthorn, Boldo, Boneset, Buckbean, Butterbur, Butternut, Calumba, Capsicum, Celery, Centaury, Chamomile, Clivers, Coltsfoot, Damiana, Dandelion, Dock, Elecampne, Eyebright, False Unicorn Root, Foxglove, Fringe Tree, Fumitory, Gentian, Ginseng, Goldenseal, Guarana, Hawthorn, Holy Thistle, Hops, Horehound, Horse Chestnut, Hydrangea, Iceland Moss, Ivy (Ground), Kava, Kola, Lavender, Lemon, Lime, Mace, Marjoram, Mistletoe, Motherwort, Myrrh, Nettle, Nux Vomica, Oak, Orange, Parsley, Peony, Pleurisy Root, Polypody, Poplar, Rhubarb, Rosemary, Sage, Sarsaparilla, Saw Palmetto, Scullcap, Stone Root, Thyme, Vervain, Wahoo, Willow, Wintergreen, Witch Hazel.

## VULNERARIES

Aloe Vera, Arnica, Comfrey, Elder, Goldenseal, Ivy (Ground), Horsetail, Marigold, Marshmallow, Myrrh, Nutmeg, Slippery Elm, St John's Wort, Witch Hazel.

# List of Latin/English Plant and Animal Names

Some manufacturers of herbal and homoeopathic medicines prefer to list the product ingredients in the classical Latin form, including the parts of the plant used.

| | |
|---|---|
| *Cortex* | bark |
| *Flos/Flora* | flowers |
| *Folium* | leaves |
| *Fruct* | fruit |
| *Herba* | flowering aerial parts of the plant |
| *Planta tota* | whole plant |
| *Radix* | roots |
| *Semen* | seeds |

## Latin/English Plant Names

| | |
|---|---|
| *Acacia senegal* | Acacia |
| *Achillea millefolium* | Yarrow |
| *Aconitum napellus* | Aconite |
| *Acorus calamus* | Sweet Flag |
| *Aesculus hippocastanum* | Horse Chestnut |
| *Agrimonia eupatoria* | Agrimony |
| *Alchemilla vulgaris* | Lady's Mantle |
| *Allium cepa* | Onion |
| *Allium sativum* | Garlic |
| *Aloe barbadensis* | Aloe Vera, Aloes |
| *Aloe ferox* | Cape Aloes |
| *Althaea officinalis* | Marshmallow |
| *Ananassa comosus* | Pineapple |
| *Anemone pulsatilla* | Pulsatilla, Pasque Flower |

| | |
|---|---|
| *Anethum graveolens* | Dill |
| *Angelica archangelica* | Angelica |
| *Angelica polymorpha* | Chinese Angelica |
| *Anthemis nobilis* | Chamomile |
| *Aphanes arvensis* | Parsley Piert |
| *Arachis hypogaea* | Arachis, Peanut |
| *Arctium lappa* | Burdock |
| *Arctostaphylos uva-ursi* | Bearberry |
| *Areca catechu* | Betel Nuts |
| *Arnica montana* | Arnica |
| *Asclepias tuberosa* | Pleurisy Root |
| *Astralagus gummifer* | Tragacanth |
| *Atropa belladonna* | Belladonna |
| *Avena sativa* | Oat |
| *Baptisia tinctoria* | Wild Indigo |
| *Barosma betulina* | Buchu |
| *Berberis vulgaris* | Barberry |
| *Betula alba* | Birch |
| *Borago officinalis* | Borage |
| *Brassica albal nigra* | Mustard |
| *Brassica napus* | Rape |
| *Bryonia dioica* | White Bryony |
| *Camellia sinensis* | Tea |
| *Capsella bursa-pastoris* | Shepherd's Purse |
| *Capsicum annum* | Capsicum |
| *Carum carvi* | Caraway |
| *Cassia acutifolia* | Alexandrian Senna |
| *Cassia augustifolia* | Tinnevelly Senna |
| *Catharanthus roseus* | Periwinkle |
| *Centaurium erythraea* | Centaury |
| *Cephaelis ipecacuanha* | Ipecacuanha |
| *Ceratonia siliqua* | Carob Bean |
| *Cetraria islandica* | Iceland Moss |

## List of Latin/English Plant and Animal Names

| | |
|---|---|
| *Chelidonium majus* | Celandine, Greater |
| *Chionanthus virginicus* | Fringe Tree |
| *Chondrus crispus* | Irish Moss |
| *Chrysanthemum cinerariaefolium* | Pyrethrum |
| *Cimifuga racemosa* | Black Cohosh |
| *Cinchona pubescens* | Cinchona |
| *Cinnamonium zeylanicum* | Cinnamon |
| *Cinnamomum camphora* | Camphor |
| *Citrus aurantium* | Neroli |
| *Citrus bergamia* | Bergamot |
| *Citrus limon* | Lemon |
| *Citrus sinensis* | Orange |
| *Cnicus benedicta* | Holy Thistle |
| *Cochlearia armoracia* | Horse Radish |
| *Cochlearia officinalis* | Scurvy Grass |
| *Cocos nucifera* | Coconut |
| *Coffea arabica* | Coffee |
| *Cola nitida* | Kola |
| *Colchicum autumnale* | Meadow Saffron |
| *Collinsonia canadensis* | Stone Root |
| *Commiphora molmol* | Myrrh |
| *Coriandrum sativa* | Coriander |
| *Cucurbita maxima* | Pumpkin |
| *Curcuma longa* | Turmeric |
| *Cydonia oblongata* | Quince |
| *Cymbopogon winterianus* | Citronella |
| *Cynara scolymus* | Artichoke |
| *Datura stramonium* | Thornapple |
| *Daucus carota* | Wild Carrot |
| *Delphinium staphisagria* | Stavesacre |
| *Digitalis lanata* | Wooly Foxglove |
| *Digitalis purpurea* | Foxglove |
| *Dioscorea villosa* | Wild Yam |

| | |
|---|---|
| *Drimia maritima* | Squill |
| *Drosera rotundifolia* | Sundew |
| *Dryopteris filix-mas* | Male Fern |
| *Echinacea augustifolia* | Echinacea |
| *Echinacea pallida* | Echinacea |
| *Echinacea purpurea* | Echinacea |
| *Elettaria cardamomum* | Cardamom |
| *Eleutherococcus senticosus* | Siberian Ginseng |
| *Elymus repens* | Couch Grass |
| *Ephedra sinica* | Ephedra |
| *Equisetum arvense* | Horsetail |
| *Eucalyptus globulus* | Eucalyptus |
| *Eugenia carophyllus* | Clove |
| *Euonymus atropurpureus* | Wahoo |
| *Eupatorium purpureum* | Gravel Root |
| *Euphorbia hirta* | Spurge |
| *Euphrasia officinalis* | Eyebright |
| *Ferula asafoetida* | Asafetida |
| *Ficus carica* | Fig |
| *Filipendula ulmaria* | Meadowsweet |
| *Foeniculum vulgare* | Fennel |
| *Frangula alnus* | Buckthorn |
| *Fragaria vesca* | Wild Strawberry |
| *Fucus vesiculosus* | Bladderwrack |
| *Fumaria officinalis* | Fumitory |
| *Galium aparine* | Clivers, Goosegrass |
| *Gaultheria procumbens* | Wintergreen |
| *Gelidium cartilagineum* | Agar |
| *Gelsemium sempervirens* | Gelsemium |
| *Gentiana lutea* | Gentian |
| *Ginkgo biloba* | Ginkgo |
| *Glechoma hederacea* | Ground Ivy |
| *Glycine soja* | Soya |

## List of Latin/English Plant and Animal Names

| | |
|---|---|
| *Glycyrrhiza glabra* | Liquorice |
| *Guaiacum officinale* | Lignum Vitae |
| *Hamamelis virginiana* | Witch Hazel |
| *Harpagophytum procumbens* | Devil's Claw |
| *Helianthus annus* | Sunflower |
| *Helionas dioica* | False Unicorn |
| *Hordeum distichon* | Barley |
| *Humulus lupulus* | Hops |
| *Hyoscyamus niger* | Henbane |
| *Hydrangea arborescens* | Hydrangea |
| *Hydrastis canadensis* | Goldenseal |
| *Hypericum perforatum* | St John's Wort |
| *Hyssopus officinalis* | Hyssop |
| *Ilex paraguensis* | Maté |
| *Inula helenium* | Elecampne |
| *Iris versicolor* | Blue Flag |
| *Jateorhiza palmata* | Calumba |
| *Juglans cinerea* | Butternut |
| *Juniperus communis* | Juniper |
| *Juniperus oxycedrus* | Cade |
| *Juniperus sabina* | Savin |
| *Krameria triandra* | Rhatany |
| *Lactuca virosa* | Wild Lettuce |
| *Larix decidua* | Larch |
| *Laurus nobilis* | Laurel |
| *Lavendula augustifolia* | Lavender |
| *Leonurus cardiaca* | Motherwort |
| *Levisticum officinalis* | Lovage |
| *Linum usitatissimum* | Linseed |
| *Lobelia inflata* | Lobelia |
| *Lycopodium clavatum* | Club Moss |
| *Lysimachia vulgaris* | Loosestrife |
| *Manihot utilissima* | Tapioca (Cassava) |

| | |
|---|---|
| *Maranta arundinacea* | Arrowroot |
| *Marrubium vulgare* | White Horehound |
| *Matricaria recutita* | Matricaria |
| *Medicago sativa* | Alfalfa |
| *Melaleuca alternifolia* | Tea Tree |
| *Melaleuca leucadendron* | Cajuput |
| *Melissa officinalis* | Lemon Balm |
| *Mentha piperita* | Peppermint |
| *Mentha spicata* | Spearmint |
| *Menyanthes trifoliata* | Buckbean |
| *Mercurialis perennis* | Dog's Mercury |
| *Myrica cerifera* | Bayberry |
| *Myristica fragrans* | Mace, Nutmeg |
| *Myroxylon balsamum* | Tolu |
| *Myroxylon balsamum var.* | Peru Balsam |
| *Nasturtium officinalis* | Watercress |
| *Oenothera biennis* | Evening Primrose |
| *Olea europaea* | Olive |
| *Origanum majorana* | Marjoram |
| *Oryza sativa* | Rice |
| *Paeonia officinalis* | Peony |
| *Palaquium gutta* | Gutta Percha |
| *Panax ginseng* | Ginseng |
| *Papaver somniferum* | Opium Poppy |
| *Parietaria diffusa* | Pellitory |
| *Passiflora incarnata* | Passion Flower |
| *Paullinia cuppana* | Guarana |
| *Pelargonium graveolens* | Geranium, Rosegeranium |
| *Petasites lybridus* | Butterbur |
| *Petroselinum crispum* | Parsley |
| *Peumus boldus* | Boldo |
| *Phytolacca americana* | Poke Root |
| *Pimenta acris* | Bay |

## List of Latin/English Plant and Animal Names

| | |
|---|---|
| *Pimento dioica* | Allspice |
| *Pimpinella anisum* | Aniseed |
| *Pinus palustris* | Southern Pitch Pine |
| *Pinus mugo var. pumilio* | Pumilio Pine |
| *Piper methysticum* | Kava Kava |
| *Piscidia erythrina* | Jamaica Dogwood |
| *Plantago ovata* | Ispaghula, Psyllium |
| *Podophyllum peltatum* | Mandrake, American |
| *Polygala senega* | Snake Root |
| *Polypodium vulgare* | Polypody |
| *Populus gileadensis* | Balm of Gilead |
| *Primula vulgaris* | Primula, Primrose |
| *Prunus amygdalus* | Almond |
| *Prunus spinosa* | Blackthorn |
| *Pulmonaria officinalis* | Lungwort |
| *Quercus robur* | Oak |
| *Ranunculus ficaria* | Pilewort |
| *Rauwolfia serpentina* | Rauwolfia |
| *Rhamnus purshiana* | Cascara |
| *Rheum officinale* | Rhubarb |
| *Rhus radicans* | Poison Ivy |
| *Rhus toxicodendron* | Poison Oak |
| *Ribes nigrum* | Blackcurrant |
| *Ricinus communis* | Castor |
| *Rosa canina* | Wild Rose, Dog Rose |
| *Rosmarinus officinalis* | Rosemary |
| *Rubus idaeus* | Raspberry |
| *Rubus villosus* | Blackberry |
| *Rumex crispus* | Yellow Dock |
| *Ruta graveolens* | Rue |
| *Salix alba* | Willow |
| *Sambucus nigra* | Elder |
| *Schoenocaulon officinale* | Sabadilla |

| | |
|---|---|
| *Scolopendrium vulgare* | Hartstongue |
| *Scutellaria lateriflora* | Scullcap |
| *Serenoa serrulata* | Saw Palmetto |
| *Simmondsia chinensis* | Jojoba |
| *Smilax officinalis* | Sarsaparilla |
| *Solanum dulcamara* | Bittersweet |
| *Solanum tuberosum* | Potato |
| *Stellaria media* | Chickweed |
| *Sterculia urens* | Indian Tragacanth |
| *Strychnos nux-vomica* | Nux Vomica |
| *Styrax benzoin* | Benzoin |
| *Symphytum officinale* | Comfrey |
| *Symplocarpus foetidus* | Skunk Cabbage |
| *Tamus communis* | Black Bryony |
| *Tanacetum parthenium* | Feverfew |
| *Taraxacum offininalis* | Dandelion |
| *Taxus brevifolia* | Yew |
| *Theobroma cacao* | Cocoa |
| *Thymus vulgaris* | Thyme |
| *Tilia platyphyllos* | Lime, Linden |
| *Trifolium pratense* | Red Clover |
| *Trigonella foenum-graecum* | Fenugreek |
| *Triticum aestivum* | Wheat |
| *Tsuga canadensis* | Hemlock Spruce |
| *Turnera diffusa* | Damiana |
| *Tussilago farfara* | Coltsfoot |
| *Ulmus fulva* | Slippery Elm |
| *Uncaria gambier* | Catechu |
| *Uncaria tomentosa* | Cat's Claw |
| *Urtica dioica* | Stinging Nettle |
| *Valeriana officinalis* | Valerian |
| *Verbena officinalis* | Vervain |
| *Vibernum prunifolium* | Black Haw |

## List of Latin/English Plant and Animal Names

| | |
|---|---|
| *Viola tricolor* | Wild Pansy |
| *Viscum album* | Mistletoe |
| *Vitex agnus castus* | Agnus Castus |
| *Vitis vinefera* | Red Vine |
| *Zanthoxylum americanum* | Prickly Ash |
| *Zea mays* | Corn, Maize |
| *Zingiber officinale* | Ginger |

## Latin/English Names of other Species

| | |
|---|---|
| *Apis mellifera* | Honey-Bee |
| *Gadus callarias* | Cod |
| *Hippoglossus hippoglossus* | Halibut |
| *Lytta vesicatoria* | Spanish Fly |
| *Ovis aries* | Sheep |
| *Perna canaliculata* | Green-Lipped Mussel |
| *Selachii* | Shark |
| *Sepiidae* | Cuttlefish |

# Bibliography

**MARTINDALE: THE COMPLETE DRUG REFERENCE**
*The Pharmaceutical Press. 33rd edition 2002.*

This book is to be found in every pharmacy in the UK and also in the reference section of libraries. It is an encyclopedia of medicines and for each entry, includes information about actions, uses, side effects, drug interactions and the brand names used throughout the world.

**THE BRITISH PHARMACOPOEIA**
*Her Majesty's Stationery Office, London.*

This provides authoritative standards for the quality of many substances and preparations (including some herbs and preparations made from them). It is a legally enforcible document in the United Kingdom, most of the Commonwealth and many other countries. Ingredients or preparations complying with the standards laid down have the letters BP after the name.

**THE BRITISH PHARMACOPOEIA CODEX**

Additional substances are included in the codex and carry the letters BPC after the name.

**EUROPEAN PHARMACOPOEIA**

This takes precedence over national standards, thus ensuring a common standard throughout the European Economic Community. The letters EP indicate compliance with the standard laid down.

## Herbal Medicines

**BRITISH HERBAL PHARMACOPOEIA**

The official publication of the British Herbal Medicine Association published to set and maintain standards of herbal medicine; it gives methods of identification, source, description of the powdered form and lays down qualitative standards. It is used mainly by manufacturers.

## POTTER'S HERBAL CYCLOPAEDIA
**Dr Elizabeth M. Williamson.**
*The C.W. Daniel Company Ltd 2003*

This invaluable book was first published in 1907 and has been reprinted many times. The current edition has been completely revised and includes extensive references for both the professional and lay reader.

## BARTRAM'S ENCYCLOPEDIA OF HERBAL MEDICINES
**Thomas Bartram, Fellow of the National Institute of Medical Herbalists.**
*Robinson Publishing Ltd 1998.*

If you wish to know more about herbal medicine, this is the book to read. Written by a herbal practitioner, it lists hundred of herbs together with actions, uses and preparations for each, plus suitable combinations. Among the A to Z of herbs, disease states are explained and herbal treatments suggested.

## HEALING PLANTS
**Lubomir Opletal and Jan Volak.**
*English edition published by Silverdale Books 2000.*

This lovely book originally produced in the Czech Republic is beautifully illustrated by Jindrich Krejca. Each herb is presented over two pages with a description of the plant, collection and preparation, active ingredients, effects and uses.

## HERBALISM
**Frank J. Lipp.**
*Macmillan Reference Books 1996.*

A less technical, highly readable book about herbs and their uses throughout the world, including folklore, healing, health and beauty, cooking and growing herbs.

## Homoeopathy

HOMOEOPATHY FOR COMMON AILMENTS
Robin Hayfield LCH.
*Gaia Books 1993.*

A useful guide for everyday problems.

THE FAMILY GUIDE TO HOMOEOPATHY
Dr Andrew Lockie.
*Hamish Hamilton for Weleda 1998.*

This is a detailed guide to homoeopathy and how the medicines can
be used to treat a wide variety of problems with complete safety.

## Aromatherapy

THE FRAGRANT PHARMACY
A Complete Guide to Aromatherapy and Essential Oils
Valerie Ann Worwood.
*Bantam Books 1990.*

Everything you need to know about essential oils and their uses,
including use in pregnancy, on babies, children and through life. Also
includes the use of essential oils in cooking and in the treatment of
pets.

## Chemistry

NATURE'S BUILDING BLOCKS An A–Z Guide to the Elements
John Emsley.
*Oxford University Press 2001.*

This wonderful book describes the elements in terms of their place
in the environment, our food, our bodies, in medicine and much more.

# Professional Associations

## Pharmacy

**The Royal Pharmaceutical Society of Great Britain.**
1 Lambeth High Street, London EC1 7JN

Established in 1841, the RPSGB maintains a register of pharmacists and of pharmacies.

A four-year university course, leading to a masters degree is followed by a one-year pre-registration training period at the end of which the society's registration examination must be passed before entry on to the register. All pharmacists are entitled to the letters MRPharmS, or FRPharmS, after their name.

## Herbal Medicine

**British Herbal Medicine Association.**
25 Church Street, Stroud, Gloucestershire GL5 1JL

The BMHA produces the British Herbal Pharmacopoeia (BHP) and various other publications on the Medicines Act relating to herbs and their uses. It does not train students for examination but works in close co-operation with the National Institute of Medical Herbalists.

**National Institute of Medical Herbalists.**
56 Longbrook Street, Exeter EX4 6AH

Established in 1864 it is the oldest and only body of professional herbalists (now known as phytotherapists) in Europe. Membership is only by examination after an approved course of study and training; a period of clinical practice must be completed before the final examination. Degree courses are available at London and Exeter universities.

All members must adhere to a professional code of ethics and are entitled to carry after their names the letters MNIHM or FNIMH.

They will supply a list of members, who are also listed in Yellow Pages.

## Homoeopathic Medicine

Many general practitioners have studied homoeopathy after qualifying as doctors, and combine conventional medicine with homoeopathy.

**The British Homoeopathic Association.**
15 Clerkenwell Close, London EC1R 0AA

**The Faculty of Homoeopathy, The Royal London Homoeopathic Hospital.**
Great Ormond Street, London WC1N 3HR

A degree course which entitles members to use the letters MFHom.

**Homoeopathic Medical Association,**
6 Livingstone Road, Gravesend, Kent DA12 5DZ

**Society of Homoeopaths**
4a Artizan Road, Northampton NN1 4HU

Holds a register of non-medically qualified homoeopaths.

Members are entitled to use the letters RSHom after their name.

## Aromatherapy

**Aromatherapy Organisations Council.**
3 Latymer Close, Braybrooke, Market Harborough, Leicester LE16 8LN

This body represents the majority of practitioners.

**International Federation of Aromatherapists.**
Stamford House, 182 Chiswick High Road, London W4 1PP

Will send you a list of registered aromatherapists, or see Yellow Pages.

# Mail-Order Suppliers

**DORWEST HERBS**
  Shipton Gorge
  Bridport
  Devon
  DT6 4LP

**HOLLAND & BARRATT DIRECT**
  PO Box 5736
  FREEPOST MID23007
  Burton Upon Trent
  DE14 1BR

**WELEDA UK LTD**
  FREEPOST 200
  Ilkeston
  Derbyshire DE7 8BR

# Index